Doubtful Dieting to Lasting Lifestyle Change

*Learn how to **lose the weight** you want, create **permanent lifestyle changes** and how to generate the **motivation** to do it*

The 6 Fundamentals to a Successful Lifestyle Change

By Devin LeBlanc

Doubtful Dieting to Lasting Lifestyle Change

This book is not intended as a substitute for the medical advice of physicians. The reader should regularly consult a physician in matters relating to his/her health and particularly with respect to any symptoms that may require diagnosis or medical attention.

ISBN# 978-0-9953275-0-4
ISBN# 978-0-9953275-2-8 (e)

Copyright © 2017 Devin LeBlanc

All rights are reserved. No part of this book may be reproduced in any form, except for the inclusion of brief quotations in review with citations, without permission in writing from the author.

Published by:
DBL Health Systems Inc.

Contact:
www.devinleblanc.com

For information, contact Devin LeBlanc at
info@devinleblanc.com

Book interior layout designing & eBook conversion by
manuscript2ebook.com

DEDICATION

I dedicate this book to all of my clients that I was lucky enough to meet over the years that allowed me to help them in their life. In doing so, you have helped me become a better coach, a better friend, and a better human being.

TABLE OF CONTENTS

Quotations 1

The Reality:
Your struggle is typical, but you can change it *now* 9

Introduction 11

Part I:
What is really holding you back from long-term
Weight Loss Success 15

Part II:
The 6 Fundamentals
- Principles to create a Successful Lifestyle Change 141

Final words 323

Thank you 325

"If I'd only known Devin 30 yrs ago and had the maturity to listen. Devin is a prince of a human being; his enthusiasm is infectious and I thank him for giving me my life back! He truly changed my life; he gave me the tools to fuel my body . . . Best of all, he gave me a lifestyle that I can maintain for the rest of my life. I have never met someone who had the education, commitment and enthusiasm to motivate me to change my entire lifestyle for the better. I genuinely believe in this lifestyle and I want all of my patients to experience the miracle that you brought to my life."

– Dr. Ken Salsman, MD

"I have always been a heavier person most of my life. I would try different diets and workouts, trying to bring my weight down to a point where I would feel better about myself. Nothing seemed to work... Eventually after spending thousands of dollars with little to no success I became frustrated and felt that this was the way I was going to be for the rest of my life... I asked Devin for his guidance and support and this has been critical for me. I

started with him at 215 lbs and I am down to 142 lbs! I can now run which I couldn't do before, and have competed in 15 different running events! I am much happier, more relaxed and positive. I am so set in my new lifestyle; I am no longer worried about my future. My life has finally changed. I would like to give Devin a special thanks, without you I would never have been able to change my life for the better."

– Melissa Halliday

"November 6th was the day I changed my life. It was the day I decided to take control of my life and that was the day I met with Devin. I weighed 402 lbs, had a 5XL shirt and wore a tight 58 inch pants. I was nervous, scared and ashamed of myself. I remember sitting waiting for my appointment, having hundreds of thoughts going through my head wondering… am I going to be able to do this?… can I lose all this weight by myself? Then I met Devin, and quickly learned I was not alone. We both knew I had a huge hill to climb so we decided to take one week at a time. Weeks turned into months and ten pounds turned into a

hundred. Devin kept me motivated by always getting me to try new things and setting small achievable goals… and eventually I lost 226 lbs. For people who read this, my advice to you is simple. Don't start tomorrow or wait until Monday, because Monday never comes… I especially want to thank Devin. Who knows where my life would be today if we never met. Thankfully because of you I can lead a life that I want to lead and not one that was lead by my weight. I'm forever grateful and you have a friend for life, and for that I say thanks! Thanks for not giving up on me, providing me with motivation and dedication and for just being a friend."

- Jeff Campbell

"I was never a big person. It wasn't until I was diagnosed with hypothyroidism that my weight was something I could no longer control. I became tired all the time and depressed about the way I looked and felt. Even being put on the medications that the doctor prescribed wasn't helping. After a few years of living like this, I began to tell myself, that this is

how it was going to be. I was going to be an overweight person, and nothing I did was going to help that. I met Devin in August, and I was a little skeptical because of trying other things and failing. Having Devin as my coach, someone that pushed me, and knew I could do it, was such a huge help. He was there to teach me more, and to show me what I could do to improve. He has changed my life forever, not only have I learned how to take care of myself, I've learned how to keep myself healthy, and feel great about the future. After going through this journey, I now know that I can do anything!"

- **Samantha Hartery**

"I am happily married and a mother of two wonderful young men. I have a wonderful life. So why did I feel as something was missing? Why did I feel as my "inner self" didn't match my "outer self"? Why? Because it didn't. I struggled to find the energy I longed to have. I felt terrible about my appearance. I made a decision to see Devin. When I reached out for Devin's help, I felt really desperate and

out of control. I feared that I would continue to "expand" until I reached 600 lbs and couldn't move. I feared that bad food would control my whole life forever. I didn't feel well and my energy levels were low. But as the weeks turned into months, and with Devin's guidance, encouragement and knowledge, I developed a routine. That routine became a lifestyle. With that lifestyle, great things happened. I continued to shrink and my energy levels continued to grow! I lost 50 wonderful pounds! I feel wonderful and confident. I love buying clothes. I finally feel "whole" – my entire "package" is complete. I realize it's not about "a diet," it's about developing a healthy lifestyle. I really owe a huge "Thank You" to Devin, I couldn't have done it without you."

– Lanie Ward

"Devin took the time for me to understand the how and the why. He also helped me come to terms with the "bad days," they will happen, that's life. The best advice I was given was "don't let a bad night become a bad weekend or month." Don't let yourself spiral down, and to

let go of the guilt and get back on track. Devin is one of the most motivating people I have ever had the pleasure to work with. He keeps me on track with positives, not negatives. "Feedback not failure," and "What did you do the next day?" are a few of my favourite quotes. I feel like I have learned so much."

– Tracy Cormier

"As a young mother of three (3, 8 & 11 years old), it was easy for me to always say "I can't eat healthy, or go to the gym, I have 3 kids!!, or "I will never be thin, I have 3 kids!!" What Devin has shown me that my kids weren't my excuse for living unhealthy, they were my reasons to live healthy! Baby weight and stretch marks are signs of motherhood, but they aren't life sentences. I always felt like I wasn't one of those "lucky" women who could have kids and a small physique, but I was WRONG! All I needed were some positive changes – a lifestyle change. Devin gave me consistency, a plan, and support. My meetings with him kept me accountable and inspired, and he believed in me, when at first, I didn't believe in myself...

and I surpassed my original weight goal in just 3 months. Yes, me a mom of 3, who faced every hardship possible – moving, financial trouble, storm damage, vehicle loss etc... I endured it, but I stayed focused and I changed my life."

– Jessica Brewster

"When I first met Devin, I knew I had found someone very professional and willing to listen as I explained to him that I am a recovering food addict. He listened to me, and assured me that he would show me a healthy way of living, one day at a time for the rest of my life. Devin has coached me and it's about achieving goals. Thank you Devin for all your help and being there… Devin has an infectious aura about him wherever he is. His positive energy shines and his book will surely motivate his readers to make healthy changes in their lives too."

– Betty LeBlanc

The Reality: Your Struggle Is Typical, But You Can Change It *Now*

Do you know someone who diets* constantly, exercises religiously and knows all that there is to know about losing weight? Have you watched as that person works diligently, trying every diet under the sun, but never experiencing long-term weight loss success? Is that person YOU?

Hello, I'm Devin LeBlanc and I help people make healthy lifestyle changes so they can stop dieting. For over 15 years, I have counselled thousands of people from all walks of life - physicians, psychologists, athletes, nutrition consultants, personal trainers, mothers, and fathers - on how to successfully lose weight and keep it off. It pains me to see someone fighting a losing battle, especially when the person tries so hard to do

---

The word "diet," "diets," or "dieting," when used in this book, are defined as restricting yourself in some way to try to lose weight - not what you eat on a daily basis.

everything right. Even health professionals are not exempt. I met and helped food coaches, dietitians, nutritionists, and personal trainers, as well as doctors, who despite improving the health of others, are unable to create that change in their lives. Why is that?

Throughout this book I will answer that question and give you all the components needed to stop dieting and to finally make the shifts needed to create lifestyle changes to lose the weight you want, for the long term. I want to help you to get off the roller coaster of crash dieting, and onto the highway on cruise control, where you rid your body of excess weight and naturally maintain your ideal weight. To do that requires a change, and this book is going to teach you how to create that change in your own life.

This book will be used as your personal blueprint to create your own path to health and wellness, through showing you how to create healthy lifestyle changes in your life so you can finally **stop trying to *lose* weight and start to get *rid* of it now.**

INTRODUCTION

Although this book is called *Doubtful Dieting to Lasting Lifestyle Change,* I will not be telling you what to eat or how to exercise. There is no specific diet or program referenced in these pages. This book is not so much a *what to do* manual as it is a *how to do it* manual.

I'll say it again: I want to help you get off the roller coaster of crash dieting and onto the highway on cruise control, where you rid your body of excess weight and naturally maintain a healthy weight. This can mean slightly different things for different people.

I am a firm believer in living healthy and happy. Personally and professionally, I know that people are never happy when they are trying to stick to the latest diet fad. So many start a diet, only to soon give up. Others, unhappy with the results of said diet, quickly turn to the next fad diet. Research has shown that most people that lose weight with any given diet, regain most of it back within a year. Does this describe you?

Over the past 15 years, I have counselled and coached over 10,000 clients in one-on-one sessions as a Transformational Health Coach. The first thing I want to tell you is **you don't need to go on another diet – you need a lifestyle change**. This is probably something that you have heard before.

Every diet plan tells you what you should or should not eat. I have made a living telling people what to eat, and even though it is extremely important, what you eat is only a small part of successful dieting. You don't need another diet: you need help realizing what stops you from achieving long-term weight loss success and the steps you have to take to make a change. You need to know how to train yourself to find the solutions that will work with YOUR unique life circumstances and not someone else's. Through my work helping thousands of successful clients, I have captured what has worked for them as well as myself to make these changes possible, and I have put what has worked in this book for you. By reading this book - you will be able to create your own personal blueprint to achieving the life and health you want – you will learn the six fundamentals to:

Get Rid of the Weight you want.

Make Permanent Lifestyle Changes in your Life.

How to Generate the Motivation to do it.

You can use this book in conjunction with any healthy, reasonable diet and exercise program. That may consist of a program you are currently on or have tried in the past or one you might want to try. The only condition is that your diet of choice is healthy and provides you with all essential nutrients for your body. You may want to discuss your diet and/or your exercise program with your health care provider.

As you go through this book, you will gather the right skills, strategies and tools necessary to make these plans work for you long term. You will also learn how you can make them a permanent part of your life. You will not just discover the means to lose those extra pounds now, but also how to keep them off permanently by learning how to make the transitions necessary to create healthy lifestyle changes.

Here's to your success,

Devin LeBlanc, BSc AHN
– Transformational Health Coach

PART I

What is Really Holding You Back From Long-Term

Weight Loss Success

THE TRUTH

Before we dive into the 6 fundamentals to long-term weight loss and a healthier you, first I must tell you the truth. You want to know the real reason why diets don't work? You might think you know, but most people do not.

The real reason why most diets don't work for long-term change is because most people don't know how to diet to make **permanent** changes. They are unclear on how to make the required shifts – not just in action, but also in thought while keeping themselves motivated. No one teaches them what to focus on, how to overcome the obstacles or how to take continuous actions to get the results they desire.

You can learn how to diet successfully. Initially, the journey is more difficult than most but the challenges that you face will become easier the more you apply the techniques of this book. Some of these ideas may seem simplistic, but they are very powerful if you appropriately apply them to your life.

I'm all about permanent changes: I'm very dedicated to helping my clients create healthy lifestyle changes and I want to do the same for you! I'm going to show you the things you need to do to get the permanent results you want. It doesn't matter if you are just starting a new healthy eating plan or if you have been dieting unsuccessfully for years. By following the principles, strategies and steps in this book, your success will become a permanent part of your life as it has for thousands of my clients.

Being in this industry for so long, I noticed that the larger part of the weight loss struggle is keeping the weight off, not losing it. I struggled myself until I found *the solution*. *The solution* is the same reason why successful clients of mine are able to maintain their weight loss. *The solution* is not about focusing on what needs to be done for the moment but for a lifetime.

Personal Struggles

I love being a coach and helping my clients create lifestyle changes to become healthier, fitter, and happier versions of themselves. But I haven't always been a coach.

Like you, I struggled with my weight. I was athletic growing up and played a lot of hockey, baseball, tennis and recreational sports. But the moment I started university, like a lot of students, I traded sports for books.

DOUBTFUL DIETING TO LASTING LIFESTYLE CHANGE

A common college term is *freshman 15,* which means that during the first year of university/college, students can put on 15 pounds. As a former athlete, I went for the gold: in my first year of university I gained 31 pounds, which is a lot, considering my 5'6 frame. And, as luck would have it, most of my weight settled right in my stomach area. (I can still remember how I felt and how low my self-esteem was at the time, and how the extra weight was even affecting my ability to study.)

But the experience also made me realize one thing: **I had to do something**. When I look back today, I know the fact that at that time both of my parents were overweight, so much so that they were considered obese was what worried me the most. I knew that if I continued on the path I was on – if I didn't do something – I was definitely heading in the same direction, and fast.

The next semester, I decided to make some changes. I didn't really know what to do, so I started with research. I was a business student, and in my spare time I studied nutrition and fitness by buying the books and magazines I could to figure out what to do. Because I had been active for most of my life, I turned to exercise first. I started to go to the school gym and even crafted a workout routine. Over the first couple months, I noticed slight differences, but I patted myself on the back for starting a weekly exercise routine and staying committed.

Next, I focused on nutrition. This is where everything changed. As I studied and started to apply what I learned, I quickly started to see the changes I wanted to see. Not just physically, but also in how I felt. Over time, I lost the weight I wanted to lose, and in the process I fell so in love with what I was learning that I switched my major from business to a science degree in Applied Human Nutrition.

I found my passion. I was acquiring knowledge that I knew would not only help me, but would help others achieve their goals and experience the same success.

During my university years, I started working in a health food store and then later managed that store and others. After graduation, I was offered a job in my field at a franchise that offered one-on-one nutrition counselling. We developed customized meal plans based on our client's goals and met with them weekly for counselling, education, accountability, and motivation. Some of our clients were there because they wanted to lose weight or manage a health condition. Others came just to be educated on how to create a healthier lifestyle for themselves.

When my boss hired me, he said that he chose me out of 40 candidates because of my overwhelming passion and energy for helping people become healthier. I was blessed for the opportunity. Later, I enjoyed what I was doing so much so that I purchased my own nutrition counselling clinic. My clientele grew rapidly, to the point where I would see nearly 50 clients per day. The business was doing great and my clients were doing even better. They were losing weight and becoming healthier. I was grateful for the opportunity to share what I had learned through my personal experience and through my education, and help clients achieve their goals and optimum health.

But, over time, I noticed something strange about my clients. Some would take what I taught them, apply it, and change their life. But sadly, most did not.

Most of my clients experienced incredible success early on: they lost all the weight they wanted to lose. But after they left, within a year, they would be right back to where they started. It puzzled me how some could keep the weight off and others could not. You could have two people in the same room and teach them the same things. One would take the information and do extremely well while the other person would do nothing, or the exact opposite.

Or, when those same clients faithfully visited me year after year, they did extremely well and met their weight loss goals. However, as soon as the regular visits stopped, they would always regain the weight.

I continually asked myself, *why?* As I searched for the answer, this started my mission to help people create sustainable, healthy lifestyle changes instead of focusing on immediate weight loss.

I initially thought that I was only teaching my clients what to eat versus teaching them the importance of exercise and the need for increased physical activity. Because I was now very active, both in and out of the gym, I knew how crucial exercise was to maintaining weight loss. So I became a certified personal trainer in order to better assist my clients. I thought this, coupled with my background in nutrition, would help my clients achieve even greater success than before. That by giving my clients personalized healthy meal plans and individualized exercise plans, this would be the cure for long-term success.

Unfortunately, I was met with disappointment: the results were the same! Nearly 100% of my clients would start out with tremendous success meeting their weight loss goals, but over time, most did not maintain their loss.

I knew that some of my clients, including myself, kept the weight off and changed their lives. But why were we the minority? I needed to know what made the difference, which intensified my research. I had to break the code, especially for my clients who worked so hard but could not manage long-term success.

Over time, and after much research and observation, I realized that the best tools in the world will not help you succeed if you are not properly positioned for success. The outward appearance of our body and the factors that construct it – from our exercise, or lack thereof, to our eating habits – are all reflections of what is going on inside. Prior to that point, the mind was one area that I had not focused on, but I learned it was the biggest factor of success. I was focused on providing all the external tools I could to equip my clients to make healthy changes instead of focusing on making changes from within.

True to form, I decided to dedicate myself to study the psychology of successful change. I was determined to understand what helped us change, how to successfully make a change, why did I change, what made some of my clients completely change, and what motivated us to change. But mostly, how to win this weight loss game from the inside out. I was relentless in my pursuit of study so that I could help my clients, and anyone I possibly could, to make permanent and healthy lifestyle changes, like I did for myself.

And, when I finally started to blend the inner rules with the outer tools of shaping our bodies, the success of my clients skyrocketed! I knew I had found the missing ingredients for lasting change. Within this book, I will share with you the six fundamentals of making a successful lifestyle change and the principles that surround them.

In Part One, I will address the importance of creating an awareness and an understanding of where you are today in your weight loss journey, and how easy it is to get stuck in the typical "dieting cycle." Part one of this book is very important, so that you can become aware of this typical cycle, and how you fit into it in your own journey. So you can create and understand how to break free from it to make a lasting change. Every successful endeavour starts with an awareness and understanding.

In Part Two, we will look at the six main fundamentals and the principles around them to make solutions for change. This is what I have discovered that all my successful clients had in common and what they did to stop their own relentless dieting to make life changes that decreased their weight permanently. Once you identify your lifetime of unhelpful habits, thoughts and actions that have held you back from success, you will need to know how to modify your lifestyle for the results you desire. Your daily routine is the reason you weigh what you do; you will learn what you need to do differently to shed your excess weight, once and for all.

MINDSET

There is always that person who has tried every diet under the sun but to no avail. Many can attest that they have no problem *losing weight*; it is *keeping the weight off* that poses the biggest problem. If you are overweight, you can probably attest to the challenge of keeping weight off versus losing it. If you think about it, anyone with a serious weight problem, has lost 100 or more pounds throughout years of dieting. Losing 10 pounds here and there, just to gain it back, then this cycle happens again and again. It pains me to see someone fight a losing battle, especially after trying so hard.

The Reason For Failure

If you are reading this, you probably are the person who is frustrated at the lack of results from all the effort that you've put in. I can safely assume that your problem is probably not a lack of knowledge about the right foods to eat or appropriate exercises to do. In fact, if you're like most people, you can probably rattle off what to do to become healthy, what foods to eat and what exercises to do. Yes, I know that you need to know how and what to eat and what to do for exercise, and some people may not know. However, in most cases, people know what to do or where to readily find that information. It's not the lack of information; it's what we do with the information that is handed to us.

We are drowning in information and starving for knowledge and wisdom.

So you probably know what to do, but do you know how to apply that information for long-term success? Can you make this a lifestyle? If you replied *yes*, why haven't you done it before now? What is stopping you?

The real challenge is your "MINDSET." If you want to make permanent changes in your life, you must master the *mindset* needed to succeed in losing and maintaining a healthy weight and lifestyle. If your *mindset* is not set for success, you may lose some weight but it will eventually return.

Maybe you are on the verge of giving up on your quest of achieving your healthy weight. Don't give up hope just yet. My work has helped over 10,000 clients successfully lose weight and become healthier. I assure you, if you follow the principles in this book, you can create a transformation in your own life.

Changing one's *mindset* is the first step to a series of changes that help you fulfill your health goals. In fact, changing one's *mindset* ensures that you maintain a healthy lifestyle long term.

Lasting change can be a reality only after we change our *mindset* towards losing weight, dieting, lifestyle, nutrition and exercise. People who struggle with their weight for years are not lazy nor do they lack the knowledge. In most cases, the repeated battle is caused by having the wrong *mindset*. If your *mindset* isn't set for success, anything you start, try, or do, will have little to no effect long term. The sad, simple truth is that all the information we gather cannot help us change our body on the outside if we don't change how we function on the inside.

The mind needs to be positioned for success before you can lose (and keep off) any excess weight. Without the right frame of mind, any weight that you do lose will come back because of the reasons we will cover later in this book.

> *Change is internal – the mind must change to ensure that the body can experience enduring change.*

A World Inside

Most of us know what needs to be done, but there is a gap between knowing and actually doing. Knowledge is valuable but means nothing if your mind is not primed to effectively use it. To become truly healthy, lose weight, and keep it off, you must first change the way you think about dieting, nutrition, fitness, and lifestyle.

Sadly, most weight loss/fitness programs pay little, if any, attention to a person's mental habits. Truthfully, one's mental habits are why most people who lose weight quickly, gain it back just as fast. Our body may do the work needed to lose weight but our mind must continue to do the work necessary to keep it off. So how do we identify what's wrong with our present *mindset*? What aspect of our habits and beliefs are working against all our efforts?

The answer to this can be found by trying to answer some simple questions about how you think and what you want. Take a moment and try to answer the following questions (be honest):

Are you getting the results you want?

Have you been struggling to lose weight?

Has the struggle been ongoing for a long period of time? Years?

Are you struggling to make healthy changes?

Does your weight fluctuate up and down constantly, although you consistently work to lose weight?

Did you answer "YES" to one or more of the above questions? Then you have just taken the first step towards becoming the person that you envision. You have understood that, even though you take effort, you are not getting the results you want, and you must do something different. The *something different* is changing your *mindset.*

Your *mindset* is the way you think about yourself, about your choices and attitudes, about your basic rules about food, exercise and about being fit. Your *mindset* dictates the diets you choose and how you implement them. It dictates not just your decisions but also your execution of these decisions.

What Is Your Mindset?

What is your *mindset*? *Mindset* includes your attitudes, perception, opinions, and more importantly, your beliefs about what you *can* achieve versus what you believe you *deserve* to achieve. Your *mindset* is the sum total of all your beliefs about yourself and about how you expect yourself to behave. It is an unconscious representation of you, your rules and your self-image.

A person's *mindset* is what drives their motivations and sets their limits. It dictates the foods you reach out for and the eating habits you have developed over your lifetime. It is what regulates the amount of exercise that you take every day.

Going beyond health, your *mindset* predicts your overall approach to life and how you respond to the twists and turns that life throws your way. Your *mindset* is comparable to a program that has been installed in your subconscious mind. It is a mental program that has almost exclusive control over your habitual behaviours.

You know, or have heard, that most people who lose a substantial amount of weight tend to gain it back within a year or two. Some may even gain more weight than they initially lost. This happens because, while they were losing weight, they did not lose their old *mindset*. Thus, the moment they stop taking the extreme effort that resulted in weight loss, they revert to old habits of eating, thinking and behaving that led to their original weight problem.

If you never fully embrace the lifestyle changes that led to your weight loss, you will soon return to the old habits that are most familiar. If you do not eventually become comfortable with the uncomfortable, you will revert back to your old habits and your weight loss will be temporary.

> *Your mindset is like a guidance system for your actions.*

Your *mindset* is like a guidance system: it governs your decisions. A lot of little decisions add up to make the habits that determine our state of health: what we prefer to eat and when; what emotions we attach to eating; the friends we have; the exercises we do and the time we spend doing them; the planning and preparation of meals at home; the choices we make when eating out as well as many others. All these factors feed into what your choices are, and subsequently, your associated body weight, health and lifestyle.

What Is Your Mindset Set For?

What is your *mindset* set for? The best way to find out is to look at your results:

Are you getting the results you want?

Is your weight always averaging around the same number?

Are you in a constant battle with your weight?

Are you constantly dieting, year after year, with little or no permanent progress?

Review your routine. What is your daily routine? Your routine will give you a clue to your *mindset*.

Most people go about their day doing the same things and thinking the same way each day. Those who are trying to lose weight will occasionally have bursts of motivation to do so.

They will start a new exercise or diet plan. Sometimes they will do both. Soon they see results and are overjoyed.

They know that the effort eventually will pay off. What they don't know is that sheer effort is not solely responsible for getting rid of excess weight and achieving optimum health. One's not-so-conscious beliefs about self, as well as a lifetime of programming – the habits we pick up and carry throughout our life – are responsible for one's long-term health. It is these beliefs and lifetime habits that drive our everyday behaviour and choices. Change starts with a change in your *mindset*.

Bonus: gunning for long term, positive changes can also help you in other areas of your life – it can make you a better worker, a better partner, and a better friend. Once you are able to understand how you are sabotaging your own efforts, you will be able to apply my principles of success in order to make you more effective, and create the *mindset* for long-term results.

Let's Go A Little Deeper: Starting Change

Having a degree in Applied Human Nutrition and being a certified personal trainer, I used to preach to my clients that living a healthy lifestyle is; 80 percent a nutritious diet and 20 percent physical activity. I still believe this is true: you have to build a healthy nutritional foundation followed by physical activity.

But, what I have truly learned after all these years of counselling and coaching clients is, long-term success hinges on your *mindset*. Your approach to your new healthy lifestyle, and the life you want to create for yourself, means EVERYTHING.

The first step is to *train the mind* to be healthy. The real problem that most people face is they have all of the know-how but don't possess the *mindset*. While I don't doubt that many people legitimately have trouble losing weight because they don't know how to *manage* their nutrition and exercise, most possess enough knowledge for successful execution.

The best solution is to change in the way they see themselves and the world around them. I now know, and believe, that it is 80 percent *mindset* and 20 percent know-how when it comes to creating a life change verses going on another diet.

Let's be realistic: how many diets have you been on in your quest for weight loss? High protein, low carb, no carb, no wheat, no dairy, no meat, all meat, shakes, supplements . . . should I go on? If nothing else, you are the expert of what *does not* work for you and what you know you *will not* do long term.

The real problem is that most people are unhappy about the "healthy" changes they make. They are waiting for their diets or exercise routines to end. A lot of this has to do with the choices they make. Instead of finding ways to make sustainable changes, people turn to extreme options which leave them feeling unfulfilled, tired, unhealthy and just waiting for the opportunity to go back to "normal." When I have a client who is in the process of losing weight say, "I can't wait until this diet is over so I can eat like I used to," I know that their days of success are numbered. He or she is still in diet mode and not committed to a lifestyle change. My job is to help them change that thinking. If you eat like you "used to," you are going to have the weight back on like you "used to". Without permanent change, your results will not be permanent.

Real change starts when you choose to improve your quality of life instead of reducing it. Since your *mindset* defines what a positive and a negative choice is, changing these basic definitions is the first step to becoming healthy.

Although you can apply this logic to any aspect of life, we will focus on health related choices, thoughts and behaviours. Changing your *mindset* means questioning the most basic ideas you have about food and exercise; fostering helpful and supportive ideas while changing destructive and counterproductive ones.

I will be honest with you – this is not an easy task. Your entire life's worth of learning fights against this change, so a new *mindset* must be implemented slowly and carefully.

Our *mindset* starts to form from our childhood experiences and the opinions and attitudes learned in various environments during the sum total of our lives. The good news is, since our *mindset* is not something we are born with but something that is learned, it is possible to unlearn these bad habits and replace them with good ones. If the appropriate methods or *principles* are applied, effective change will result.

Cognitive Behavioural Therapy (CBT)

Some of the seminal work in changing deep rooted thoughts and beliefs, has been done by psychologists who developed what is known as Cognitive Behavioural Therapy (CBT). This branch of psychological therapy was formed when counsellors and therapists realized that a lot of our actions are rooted in old beliefs that we are often unaware of.

When we learn beliefs and choices that hinder our growth, we self-sabotage. The only way to counter this tendency is to change the basic thought and beliefs of the individual. Our thoughts lead to our feelings that lead to our actions which then lead to the results that we are getting. Over time, these repeated actions become habits. But why do we think the thoughts we think? That is our *mindset* in action. So knowing this, we can rewrite it as follows:

> *Our mindset leads to our thoughts which leads to how we feel which leads to our actions which gives us our results.*

Throughout this book, we will apply principles to consciously alter our destructive, self-sabotaging thoughts and behaviours while applying more constructive, helpful ones. For over a decade, I have applied these principles to help my clients achieve the long-term results they wanted. If you are ready to put in the effort, I can help you achieve the same results using the same process.

Your Mindset = Your Weight Set Point.
All of us have a hidden set point for our weight:

When people come to see me and I talk about changing their *mindset*, they are confused. They believe that they have already changed their *mindset* by deciding to lose weight and walking into my clinic. But, unfortunately, this is not usually the case.

The real problem is that most people's *mindset* is programmed for dieting instead of a lifestyle change. It is programmed to lose weight, not get rid of weight or gain optimum health.

While it is important to lose excess weight, it is more important to achieve a healthy weight and maintain a healthy lifestyle long term. Often we are so seduced by quick, short-term results that we do not plan for long-term success. We just look at obtaining results and don't put much thought into the process.

> *No plans for long-term success =*
> *guaranteed failure*

DOUBTFUL DIETING TO LASTING LIFESTYLE CHANGE

We need to change our perspective from the near to the distant future; in order to do so, we must examine our distant past. This past will help you know why you are at your present weight and will help you to realize what has upset your health along the way.

Your Mindset = Your Weight Set Point. All of us have a hidden set point for our weight: an internal point that regulates our weight and keeps it within a certain range. This is why most people hit a plateau quickly when they start to lose weight – their *mindset* is working against them.

The set point is why you start to lose motivation or crave *forbidden foods* early on in your diet. You can deploy every exercise and diet trick there is, but unless you can convince your body to change its weight set point, all the tips and tricks in the world won't give you the lasting impact you desire.

Why is it so hard to change your weight set point? This is because it is governed by your unconscious *mindset*. It is like an internal thermostat for your weight: when your weight fluctuates or goes beyond a "comfortable" level, your weight set point is activated. If you have suddenly gained enough weight to make you feel uncomfortable, you will do whatever it takes to lose that weight until you feel comfortable again.

The same thing will happen when you lose weight. Unconsciously, if you lose a large portion of weight that you are not used to having off your body, even if you are in a healthy weight range, subconsciously you will sabotage yourself to put that weight back on.

Coach Devin, you ask, *if that's true, why can people slowly gain so much weight over their lives*? Because the weight set point can be fooled. It worries about sudden changes, and with age and slow lifestyle changes, it continuously increases one's weight little by little each year.

As you study and review this book, remember this is not a quick fix or short-term strategy. This is not a chance to blame external factors for your present weight. The principles and processes we will partake in assign no blame to anyone. Rather, they try to understand the circumstances that created a misfit between your *mindset* and your needs. You have to change your *mindset* to change your weight set point.

But how is a winning *mindset* formed? What actions need to be repeated for success? And, once you identify the winning *mindset*, how do you acquire, retain and maintain it?

In this book, I will help you identify and change problematic thoughts, feelings and actions you are currently taking. I will then share valuable, supportive, healthy and more effective ones for you to replace the old with. This process is not about denying yourself the things that you love; it is about changing your approach to how you incorporate those things while achieving your lifestyle goals for the rest of your life.

How is your *mindset* formed? Repetition of information and actions. How do you change your *mindset?* By repetition of information and actions.

It is about being healthier as well as happier in the long run. If you are ready to invest in yourself and put in the time, we will continue on what will be a fulfilling and rewarding journey.

CONDITIONED

We eat to satisfy our hunger but we overeat to satisfy the mind.

Have you reached for some food even though you were not hungry? Maybe an unhealthy night snack when you were trying to avoid eating at night. Most people do this without even thinking.

Let me ease a bit of your pain: partially, it is not your fault. Our eating and exercise habits, or lack thereof – what we eat or don't; the choices we make to eat to live or eat to fill a void; the choice to repeat destructive habits that we know work against us but seem powerless to control – are all programmed since you were young. The old cliché holds much weight when it comes to your attitude regarding a healthy lifestyle: *we are a product of our environment*. (I'll elaborate shortly.)

Many of my clients come to me because they are frustrated with their attempts to lose weight. Most of them have habits that encourage them to pick at food, look for certain types of food at certain times (even when they are not hungry), and to overeat certain meals while not having enough at others. These are programmed habits that motivate them to eat in certain ways even when they are trying not to. The sad part? Consciously they may not even be aware of what they are doing.

Once they visit me, they become more aware of what they are eating and what their portions should be. They become aware of what prompts their snacking. I usually hear responses like, "I am not hungry at night, I just want to eat." This desire to eat is ruled by their mind, not their stomach. Often, they have full bellies but crave some kind of comfort/snack food.

Why Does Food = Comfort?

Why, for some, does food equate to comfort? This is the perfect example of mental programming – the belief that eating will make us feel better. While a lot of it comes from old habits, there are so many other factors that fuel "comfort food."

> Example: You are tired at the end of the day and a decadent treat cries out to your emotions and taste buds. While you relax, your brain also takes a break and this decadent treat becomes even more appealing. And then, you

turn on the T.V., you are plagued by multiple food advertisements that are almost hypnotic, and trigger even more cravings that didn't exist before.

The opposite is also true: once you give in and try to satisfy those cravings, you find the "comfort food" wasn't as comforting as you anticipated. So often, we turn to some form of comfort food, even though we know it's not good for us or our goals, only to be disappointed. Many times, what seems good at first bite, leaves us dissatisfied and plagued by guilt. You have just derailed your healthy diet for nothing. Now I know that, while creating healthy lifestyle changes, you will have a "treat" here and there. What I'm talking about is when those treats are habitual and unplanned which takes you further away from your health goals.

So why do we continue to repeat this destructive behaviour over and over again? Why don't we just stop and opt for healthier alternatives? The answer can be found in our programming or the influence of learned behaviours.

Our *mindset* towards food is governed in many ways by what we saw, heard, experienced and ate while growing up. What we learned and saw around us, feeds our attitudes and options about food and our food and exercise choices. On the other hand, what and how we ate as children and what made us feel better back in the day, forms the basis of our food preferences today. Even the situations where we reach for comfort food, are unknowingly influenced by our past experiences.

A person's state of mind is the source of their life experience, and thus, their performance.

We are rarely aware of any of this. To our conscious mind, our food choices and habits are influenced by situational factors. Erroneously, we tend to believe that we can control these. But a lot of the factors that really influence our food choices, are not even ours.

The driving influencers of our food choices are derived from the ideas, preferences and attitudes of leading figures in our childhood. Our parents, grandparents, siblings, friends, teachers and even media – radio, TV and advertisements we saw as children – play a role in influencing our choices and preferences.

Finding The Source

You have to look back in your past and ask yourself, *how did those close to me influence me?* A very important step towards changing your *mindset* and your food habits, is to take a moment and understand the influences that shaped your attitudes and behaviours towards food and health.

For example, take some time to reflect. Consider the choices and behaviours of your parents and of the other people who influenced you. How did your parents eat? What were their attitudes and opinions about dieting and weight? Did they exercise or play sports? Did they encourage you to exercise?

You may find that the attitudes and habits that your parents had, greatly influenced yours. You may find yourself repeating their choices, or you may find that you have habits that are vastly different from theirs.

If your parents were active and focused on physical fitness, you may find yourself gunning for the same. On the other hand, if they preferred snacking at night and encouraged large portions at meals without demonstrating the importance of exercising regularly, you may find yourself doing the same. Do you reach for large portions of comfort food without thinking? Is exercise a little or nonexistent part of your life?

The opposite can also be true. You may find that your choices greatly differ from what was demonstrated before you. For example, perhaps you had a strict diet as a child which makes you crave rich, unhealthy foods today. Or maybe you learned to associate food with guilt and unhealthy eating is a secret pleasure for you.

Think back to your own experience as a child. Did you struggle with weight as you grew up? Did your parents struggle with their weight? Were you ever asked to lose or gain weight or were you discouraged from focusing on your body? Did you try diets when growing up? Did you see your parents going on diets? Did you see your weight yo-yo?

If weight was an issue that received constant attention in your home, more than likely that has influenced your attitudes about weight loss or created health anxieties. Too often, children can be asked to eat more than their hunger levels to satisfy the character and emotions of adults. This eventually becomes a habit. Parents may unknowingly be sending their children conflicting messages to stay fit and healthy but also to eat in excess. This combination yields a lifelong struggle to eat everything put in front of you while simultaneously attempting to stay fit.

Friends also play a very important role in the habits we form and how we see ourselves. Friends often influence our ideas and attitudes more than adults do when we are growing up.

We learn a lot of what we expect to look like and behaviours from our friends. We pick up habits that help us fit into a group and these habits often follow us into adulthood. Adolescents also learn dieting from their friends and these friends help shape their opinions and preferences.

Take this opportunity to recall your personal experiences with weight. Did you ever try to lose weight? If so, what did you do? Did you have a dramatic experience growing up that made you turn to food? Were you taught to think of food as fuel and nourishment, or as a source of pleasure, as a treat or as something bad? Did you ever think of food as your friend or enemy? Were you taught about what is unhealthy versus healthy ways of eating?

Culture can also play a big role in your eating. What did your culture teach you about food? Do you still follow the same principles, or have you deviated from them?

Knowing *what* you associate different foods with will help you understand *why* you eat in a certain way or crave certain foods over others. You'll discover why you have trouble controlling your portions and what you eat and why you might be resistant to trying something new.

A Life Time Of Learning

Keep asking yourself questions to find out how your ideas about weight, food and exercise developed across your lifetime. Take some time, if necessary, to make sense of your memories; be honest with yourself. This will reveal how you were conditioned or programmed from a young age to have the *mindset* and habits that you have today.

I have developed a series of exercises to help you identify some of the roots of your habits today. Please answer each question as honestly as you can. To assist you, I will give examples from my own life as well as the lives of some of my clients.

Let's start with a simple one: ***When you were growing up, what did you hear that could have shaped your ideas and opinions when it comes to your eating?*** Some of the most popular statements commonly heard are:

You have to have something sweet to finish a meal.

Finish your supper or you can't go out to play.

If you want to lose weight, you need to starve yourself.

You are what you eat.

Healthy food is not supposed to taste good (or be fun).

Perhaps a piece of cake and ice cream for dessert will make you feel better.

Food is how people show love; the more I feed you, the more I love you.

Healthy eating is boring and tasteless.

Diet food is food not meant to be enjoyed.

Sound familiar? Most people have heard these conflicting messages. You can probably think of a lot more that pertain to your life growing up. A lot of us have been conditioned to associate comfort food with love and happiness and healthy things with being unhappy.

Many of these statements come from my own childhood. I know that my mother and other adults meant well and repeated what they learned from their childhood. But, for a young impressionable mind, these ideas become the catalyst for which unhealthy adult lifestyle choices are made.

Similarly, a lot of other "innocent" experiences can make a strong impact on one's adult lifestyle choices. Think about each of the questions below in the same way that we tackled the last one regarding your upbringing.

The first set of questions had to do with the things you *heard* growing up and that you learned from the experiences and opinions of others. The second set has to do with what you *saw* growing up and maybe became habits you formed because of the rules given to you with respect to food and exercise.

As you go through the list you will see how the experiences of others, coupled with your own as a child, slowly formed your current *mindset* about food, exercise, and health. Remember, we are not trying to assign blame to anyone but trying to understand the unique set of circumstances that have guided you to your present *mindset*.

What did you <u>see</u> around you while growing up?

A lot of healthy or unhealthy eaters?

Frequent and consistent exercise or no additional exercise?

Food items that you instantly said you disliked before even tasting it? If so, why?

When viewing the habits of someone "dieting," what results did you see?

Did you see others around you encouraged to eat a certain way, certain foods or a certain quantity, to demonstrate love and affection?

What were the eating patterns of those around you? Did you see your family eating breakfast or having snacks after supper? Did you see them eat 3 meals a day? Or did they eat more or less than that? What were the portions like?

What television shows and movies did you watch? How did they shape your ideas about food?

What did you *do* growing up around eating/exercising?

Did you have to finish your full plate, (regardless of whether you were hungry or full), before you had dessert or were allowed to leave the table?

How many meals did you eat a day? Did you snack? When?

Did you exercise?

Did you eat home cooked meals or a lot of quick processed foods?

Did you learn how to cook at a young age?

Did you eat out a lot? Or did you eat at home a lot?

DOUBTFUL DIETING TO LASTING LIFESTYLE CHANGE

Did you "diet?"

Did you and your family eat at the table for meals?

Were you in the habit of eating – things like popcorn, candy or chips – every time you watched a movie or a certain TV program?

Was food a symbol of joy in your household or used as a source of comfort? Was it both?

While the above list is long, I can hardly call it *exhaustive*. You probably have many personal experiences that you can add to this list. Actually, I encourage you to do so.

Below, list your observations, from your childhood and beyond, what you can remember that demonstrate your ideas about food and health.

In your childhood, as it relates to healthy eating and exercise, what did you…?

	See	Hear	Do
1	_____	_____	_____
2	_____	_____	_____
3	_____	_____	_____
4	_____	_____	_____
5	_____	_____	_____

Changing The Message

If you are a parent, or regularly work with children, you want to also consider what messages you are passing onto them. Use your awareness of how the statements from your childhood shaped your relationship with food and exercise. Make changes, where necessary, when it comes to what you pass onto the next generation.

Maryann Jacobsen, MS, RD, is a registered dietitian who has done extensive work on how to teach children to eat well. She shares a lot of her findings on her website (*http://www.raisehealthyeaters.com*) as well as what we can say to change the message. Here are some of the more common ones:

You say: "You didn't eat enough. Take a few more bites and then you can leave the table."

The child hears: "Mom/dad/adult knows when I'm full versus my body telling me that I am."

Say instead: "Make sure you got enough to eat because the next meal won't be until _____ (breakfast/lunch/dinner/snack time)." This gives the child a clear indication that they have to fuel up for a particular period and allows them to judge for themselves how much is enough.

You say: "If you eat some of your veggies, you can have dessert."

The child hears: "Vegetables must be suffered through to get the good stuff – dessert!" (A child who internalizes this is likely to start looking for a chance to skip vegetables since they now represent boring food.)

Instead: Instead of nagging and offering comfort food as a reward, offer tasty vegetables and often. Find exciting ways to cook nutritious vegetables and model healthy eating.

You say: "See, X is eating it, why don't you?" *When it comes to eating a new healthy food.*

The child hears: "X is a better eater than I."

Say instead: "You will learn to appreciate it, dear. It takes time and many tries before we learn to like a new food."

You say: "Good job!" (This occurs normally after eating.)

The child hears: "Mommy and daddy are proud of me when I eat more food." This prompts the child to eat more in order to gain more praise. This also conditions him or her, even as an adult, to finish food just because it is on their plates.

Say instead: "You always do a good job eating when you listen to your tummy."

You say: "If you are good in the store, you can have a cookie." Or, "If you don't stop doing that, you won't get any ice cream tonight."

The child hears: "Every time I'm good, I'll get a treat!" In adulthood, this could lead to a pattern of self-rewarding with rich foods that cause havoc with any attempt to lose weight.

Instead: Let your child know, ahead of time, the consequences that will happen if he or she misbehaves – leave food out of it.

What I Learned About Food As A Child….

Let me help you make sense of your own experiences by sharing mine. When I was a child, my parents and grandparents had certain attitudes and habits associated with eating. Those attitudes and habits made a big impression on me: my childhood memories of my grandparent's home were largely connected to food.

While they were living, my grandparents filled their home with food. Despite not having a lot of money, my grandparent's house always had plenty of food. Whenever we would visit, I felt like royalty with the overabundance of food that was prepared. Because my grandmother loved to bake, I remember an array of 13 different desserts one Christmas – 13!

Of course, every spread was not so elaborate, but there was always so much food at every meal that it was physically impossible to enjoy all the choices in one sitting. Every meal course included baked items, breads and sweets, in addition to the main selections.

To add to this breeding ground of unhealthy eating, my grandmother was a firm believer in multiple helpings. She would not let us get up without having a second helping, if not a third, of every course! Overeating was practically mandatory and we were all fed until we burst at the seams.

Anyone who tried to leave the table before indulging in at least two plates of everything, would be asked questions like, *"Why don't you want some more? Don't you like my cooking?"* I must say that she was a wonderful cook and we all adored her food. But our enjoyment was not enough; my grandmother was not satisfied until we demonstrated our love by overeating. To her, food was a sign of love, so the moment you stepped into her house, she would force you to eat something.

This habit of hers had a lot to do with some of my grandfather's experiences as a young man. My grandfather was in the Army during World War II. He was captured and held as a prisoner of war (POW) in Germany for a year and a half until his release at the end of the war.

While he was a prisoner, my grandfather was forced to work in the fields and prepare the produce for the meals of the prisoners and guards. It was hard work and the prisoners were fed just enough to keep them alive. My grandfather would tell us how he survived by sneaking some food when he could to keep him going in the fields. He would also eat discarded foods that he had to clean, like carrot tops and potato skins to keep up his strength.

This experience left him dramatically underweight and malnourished; he went from being 176 pounds at the beginning of the war to 117 pounds when he returned home. Of course, he developed other health issues with his POW experience as did countless others.

Upon my grandfather's return, appalled by her husband's condition, my grandmother vowed that he would never go hungry again. Both my grandfather and grandmother gained a tremendous respect for food; it became a way to care, to show love and to provide comfort. Overeating started to become a way of life for them.

My father, who was a child at this time, grew up in this environment of overeating. As a consequence, overeating became a habit for him, and he has battled weight issues and obesity for most of his adult life.

My mother's family had a different story but it ended the same. My mother's father was a fisherman so he worked from daybreak to dusk for eight months of the year. My grandmother, who had no way of reaching him once he had left the house, would always welcome him at the end of the day with a big feast ending in dessert. That was my grandmother's way of showing her husband how much she missed him.

My mother recalls how my grandmother – who was well known for her baking skills, especially her pies – would make three fresh pies every week and they had to be finished within the week. My mother also recalls how she would have a small breakfast and lunch followed by heavy suppers always ending with sweets. This was a habit that my grandfather maintained all his life. He didn't consider the meal finished without his sweet or dessert after his supper.

My parents, who grew up around so much food, carried the majority of the unhealthy lifestyle patterns learned into their adulthood. As a child, I remember all the heavy suppers followed by something for your sweet tooth. We ate in front of the TV regularly. I also remember having to finish all of my very generous helpings before I was allowed outside to play. As a result, I quickly learned to overeat.

Of course, with the constant stream of cookies and pies around also, late night snacking was widely accepted and practiced. Thus, by the time I reached university, I was in the habit of eating a light breakfast (if any), and lunch (if any), followed by a very heavy dinner and a lot of late night unhealthy snacking.

I can remember that I would eat so much at the end of each day, that I would fall asleep with a full belly, only to wake up drowsy with no desire to eat in the morning. I call this, waking up with a *food hangover*. Has this after happened to you? This became my habit. As I grew older, my weight increased. It would take years of research, training, failures and hard work, before I learned how to reverse this downward spiral and to be able to give back and to teach others what to do and how to do it.

> ***And, this is how I know that you can too. If you go about it the right way.***

The Force Of Habits

90 to 95 percent of what you do is based on your habits. Hopefully you are now convinced that your weight is a result of your inter-programming. If you are unsure of whether you have unhealthy, self-sabotaging habits, take a look at your results, your weight. If you are not at a healthy weight, you need to examine your habits. The outside, your body, is a total reflection of what is going on the inside.

What are your current food and exercise habits?

Are you programmed to be active or inactive?

Are you programmed to eat breakfast or to eat heavy meals at night?

What are your portions like?

Do you snack instead of eating balanced meals?

Do you eat out a lot or do you encourage preparing your meals at home?

Do you plan meals ahead of time or on the go?

What is your automatic responses to negative or positive emotions around food?

Are you now seeing trends in your behaviour that are sabotaging your efforts? Are you becoming aware of the conditioning and programming that makes you eat in ways that may work against you and your success? Do you realize that you eat certain things out of habit? Somewhere along the way, has your mind and body forgotten how to gauge the amount you need to eat? Or have you started triggering impulsive eating to please other people? Are you becoming aware of your helpful and unhelpful habits as well as their origin?

If you answered *yes* to any of the above, congratulations! You have just had a breakthrough that can move you ahead in forming healthy, useful habits while consciously changing the unhelpful ones. This awareness will help you identify problem areas in your own conditioning that you will need to address in order to create newer, healthier habits, that will bring you to where you want to be.

COMFORT ZONE

In the last couple of sections, we discussed the factors that contribute to the formation of our *mindset*. We now know that our childhoods, the habits and attitudes of the people around us and our own experiences, all lead to the development and strengthening of our *mindset*. Now that you have had the opportunity to explore your past, let's see what factors in our current environment play a major role in our *mindset* and health behaviours.

Our Mental Process

Our *mindset* acts like a filter, so it is a key factor in which thoughts we choose to entertain. One's *mindset* establishes our expectations from ourselves and from our environment. It informs us of how we should interpret different situations and what to think – when, what or where to eat or exercise.

These thoughts in turn influence our feelings. Our thoughts are interpretations of our experiences and of the things we encounter. These interpretations lead us to feel in ways congruent to our experiences. For example, when we see our reflection and think, "*I look good,*" we feel happy and confident. But when we look at the reflection and think, "*I look fat,*" we feel unhappy, dejected and maybe even angry with ourselves.

Next are our emotions. Emotions influence our actions by motivating us to carry out specific tasks. Positive emotions motivate us to do things that will help us continue to feel good. Negative emotions motivate us to do things that will reduce the extent to which we act and react. Without our emotions, our actions would feel purposeless.

All our actions and choices culminate into the results we see. If we have been motivated to carry out healthy activities, like eating healthy meals and exercising regularly, then we see ourselves becoming healthy. But if we have been responding to motivations that have led us down unhealthy paths, like eating unhealthy foods and snacks regularly, than we see ourselves becoming heavier and less fit.

If we carry out the same actions for long enough, they solidify into our habits and become what we automatically practice (or do). Our habits are not built on the basis of what is good or bad for us; they are built on the basis of what we have learned to want and not want. Thus, many people who know they have unhelpful health habits, still find it very difficult to break them. After all, there are a number of processes that have lead up to the habits and expectations that they have.

If a habit has been practiced long enough, it becomes a part of your comfort zone – the thoughts, emotions, preferences, behaviours and beliefs that are automatic. This automation controls most of our unconsciously motivated behaviour – those factors that define the "safe" and "convenient" responses for one's self.

Your comfort zone helps keep you safe by allowing you to do things that are proven to not harm you (immediately). On the other hand, it excludes all the thoughts, actions, emotions and motivations that are unfamiliar to us. It makes us suspicious of these unfamiliar experiences and strives to dissuade us from going down potentially new and risky paths.

Since so much of what we think, feel and do is governed by our comfort zone, it is only natural that our weight, at any given time, is also influenced by our comfort zone. Our bodies know what a familiar weight is and strives to maintain it against all odds. All the habits of our comfort zone come together to influence our choices, which in turn regulate and maintain our set weight.

Basically, whatever you think will affect your emotions; whatever you feel will guide your behaviour. Your behaviour can predict the results you see. Over time, your consistent behaviours will become your habits. Your comfort zone is a collection of your habits, and without even realizing it, you are stuck in a loop that plays out over and over again.

Dieting

Many people have mastered the art of dieting. They try every new gimmick that their friends tell them about or they read or see on an infomercial. Although many diets do yield short-term results, most are not sustainable.

The moment one stops following the diet – either because the period is over, interest is lost, or the degree of difficulty in fitting it into one's current lifestyle – all weight lost comes back and often with additional pounds.

Unfortunately, short term or inconsistent dieting, often is part of our comfort zone. In reality, this is one of the reasons we feel so trapped and helpless. We feel like we are doing everything we can but are not able to obtain long-term weight loss. Every time we lose a little weight after a diet, we feel great; every time it comes back, we feel dejected.

It does seem counter intuitive, but this habit of dieting is what may be preventing you from making suitable life changes. It traps us in a never-ending loop by giving us short-term hopes and results. Any habit is difficult to change. This is basically because it feeds a certain need, even if only temporarily. Secondly, the habit is comfortable and familiar, which makes change even more difficult. Since our habits are developed from our past experiences and conditioning, they can be incredibly resistant to change.

But change really is possible; if we know the right ways to implement it.

We don't resist *change*; we resist *being changed*. Most of us want change but we don't want to put in the effort required to change. Wanting change is typically not the problem. It's the change we have to ensure, from the inside out, that we resist. The change we resist is not so much in taking new actions but in our *mindset* and in our comfortable habits.

People may think it is easier to take new actions – to form a new habit versus changing an old one. The reality is, you cannot just create a new habit without replacing an old one. *If that's true*, you ask, *how do we implement lasting, deep reaching change?* The first question on this path is, *do you really want to change? Yes I do*, many of you will reply. That desire for change is what brought you to this book.

I know that you are looking to make changes to your habits that will help you get in the shape you want, lose excess weight and become an overall healthier person. Just like the clients I see every day, you also want to turn things around so that you can achieve your health goals and maintain them.

The next question then is, *why hasn't that change happened for you?* By now you know the answer to that – you have been limited by your *mindset* and habits rooted in your comfort zone. Most of us want the desired change in our lives but we don't want to make overreaching changes in the way we live.

We start a new diet and exercise program but we don't feel that we are seeing the results of our actions. The truth, my friend, is you are receiving the fruit of your actions and not the ones you think.

We don't resist functional change; we resist a change to our attitudes and beliefs and the comfortable habits we have had for most of our lives. And this is understandable. We resist this change because we are comfortable with these aspects of our lives. If we weren't so accepting of the way we think and feel we wouldn't practice it as often.

Many of us are also blind to these comfort zones, since they have been a part of our lifestyle for so long. Often, people don't even realize that these comfort zones are sabotaging their fitness, nutrition, health, and weight goals. They don't see the connections between these old habits and attitudes and their present health challenges. But, the fact is, our habits, comfort zones and attitudes do indeed determine how healthy we are and the choices we make about our health. Thus, we are often "comfortable" in the way we think and live, but are not truly happy. The sad truth is that we can be "comfortable" but miserable.

There is no doubt that you desire to live a healthier lifestyle and to lose weight; it is evident from the effort you take. But this effort is ineffective because you are unwittingly resisting deep, major change. Let's take a look at the effort that you do take. Often, it involves slight change or additional effort but does not result in major lifestyle changes.

DOUBTFUL DIETING TO LASTING LIFESTYLE CHANGE

Maybe you buy the latest "magic diet pill." This fat burning pill poses no major disruption in your lifestyle, takes minimum effort and little to no change.

Or perhaps you prefer a 15-day or 30-day cleanse or detox diet. This certainly takes more effort and requires you to change your food choices during the duration of the cleanse. But you power through because the change is for a limited period of time.

You count the days and push yourself to complete the course, especially once you start seeing the weight loss. The problem with this is two-fold – there are no long lasting results and the weight soon returns. Second, many of these diets can be unhealthy and deprive the body of essential nutrients. So, the miracle cleanse or detox diet can actually work against you as far as long-term weight loss is concerned. Don't get me wrong, I do think some "cleanses" are healthy, and it could also be a great gateway for you to continue with a healthy lifestyle after the initial cleanse. What I'm referring to is going on a cleanse or detox diet for a short time just for weight loss.

Most of the diets out there are not realistic on a long-term basis. But since they give us short-term weight loss results, we are fooled into following them again and again. The first step in ridding yourself of them is to recognize that, not only is the diet not a permanent part of your lifestyle, the associated weight loss isn't either. All the weight we lose returns once we go back to our regular lifestyle.

We need to stop focusing on the temporary changes and start thinking about sustainable, permanent ones. So the first thing you have to ask yourself before starting any program or diet is, *to the best of my knowledge, is this healthy? And… is this livable?*

The Weight Zone

Our weight zone, or the typical weight we tend to maintain, is determined by our comfort zone. When we realize that we are gaining weight, we become uncomfortable and try to get our weight back to a point where we feel comfortable.

That 10 pounds gained may go away after a month long diet, but once we feel more comfortable, we tend to take less action towards losing weight. The moment we are comfortable with our weight, old habits start coming back. Now, since these are the same habits and the same comfort zone that caused the weight gain in the first place, we slowly start gaining weight and are right back to where we started.

Question The Comfort

Let's start the process of permanent change by accepting that our comfort zone is the reason why we weigh what we weigh. If this is true, how can we sustain weight loss by any means without changing our comfort zone? You can not. To permanently change your weight, you must change your comfort zone. You have to start to do *new things* to start to receive *new results*. This process may take a little time and mental effort, but we are looking for long term and self-sustaining results.

How do you start to change your comfort zone? You start by making choices outside of your current comfort zone that will bring you closer to the lifestyle and results you want. Choices like joining that fitness class, or learning to cook in healthy ways or finding out and implementing healthy portions for you. Once you have this awareness, you have to apply that knowledge to your daily routine *consistently*.

Once you continue to make these new choices outside of your current comfort zone, you will not only lose weight and become fit, over time you will continue to stay fit by eventually creating a new comfort zone around these new choices. And when you are healthier and more fit, you will have established a new comfort zone that is invaluable to your long-term success. But this takes time.

Something that I have seen with many of my clients is, without knowing it, they sabotage their own efforts when they are trying to lose weight. For most people, their comfort zone habits are useful in dealing with the everyday small ups and downs. But once they start losing weight, the demand for continued effort makes their everyday choices less comfortable.

They start to doubt their own efforts and see weekly weight loss as "too good to be true." So they unwittingly self-correct and sabotage their efforts. As stated earlier, the opposite is also true. When they gain weight, they also feel uncomfortable since they are deviating from their set comfort zone and comfortable weight zone. So when they start to gain weight, they get uncomfortable and try to get rid of the extra weight.

The take away from this is, if we can overtime reset our comfort zone and establish new habits, we can naturally support a healthy weight set point. Before long, these new habits become second nature to maintaining a healthy weight.

Why Do We Cling To Our Comfort Zone?

Because it is *comfortable*. *Comfortable* is not the same as healthy or even helpful. People find it difficult to move out of their comfort zone, forgetting that it is entirely of their own choosing. They maintain inaccurate beliefs about themselves and harbour self-doubt. These negative images, negative self-talk and pre-programmed comfort zones always seem to cancel out their good intentions, regardless of how hard they try.

At times like this, your comfort zone is like a large and comfortable, self-made prison. For someone who does not recognize how this can be limiting, it is as if they built the walls of this prison and threw away the key.

All of the mistaken beliefs we have about ourselves – about food, health and fitness – become knit together to lock us into a prisoner-like state. All the expectations that we picked up from our families and our friends, all the compulsions that we impose on ourselves without realizing the costs, they all stop us from evoking real change.

Your next question will be, *"How do I recognize these limiting beliefs?"* The answer is quite simple: *by looking at what is limiting your success*. Exactly what stops you from getting the results you want to achieve?

Start questioning your beliefs and how they affect your diet and exercise choices. Listen to your language. Statements starting with "I can't" or "I should" are limiting. These statements join together and serve to keep you from achieving and maintaining your health goals.

Any healthy choices qualified with a "but" also limit our actions. For example, the statement "I will drink 2 liters of water every day," will help you feel better and be healthy. But when you add to that statement, ". . . but, if I have company over or when family visits, I may not . . ." you are setting yourself up for failure through inconsistency which weakens these habits.

Any limiting beliefs are directly connected to your past; to overcome and create a new change or result, you must think outside your comfort zone. You must set aside your limiting beliefs to open the door to make positive changes in your life. This is where your *mindset* will start to change which initiates transformation.

Fearing Fear

New is exciting but it is also *scary*. The old way may be unhealthy but it is *comfortable* and *known*. Thus, when you are trying to establish new habits, realize that you are fighting against a natural fear of the new and unknown. Even if you arm yourself with all the knowledge in the world, your responses – including your emotions after making new choices or your experiences thereafter – are all part of the great unknown.

When we encounter unfamiliar experiences, our minds instantly seek out known, comforting experiences. Because old norms are so well known, they can cancel out the present, good intentions if we are not vigilant. You must stay alert, aware, and consistent, when making new healthy choices. This is daily work so past, unhealthy habits don't return. This is part of the struggle to keep new habits, making it imperative that we completely change our *mindset* in order to experience optimum health and maintain it.

Eternal Optimism

Human beings are essentially optimistic people. We want to see the silver lining to dark clouds and we want to look for the rainbow after torrential rains. Thus, even after a number of failed dieting attempts or weight regain, we approach each new diet as "the one" that will finally give us the results we desire. We put past disappointment behind us and expect the best results from this new, magic pill or quick fix diet.

In doing so, we not only start off the journey to another failure, but often sabotage our overall health for the sake of temporary weight loss. It doesn't help that media and friends are hyping up this new pill or diet and the so called "success stories" heighten our sense of failure when we don't get the results we wanted.

Our brain is designed to *survive* not to *thrive*. While long-term changes seem reasonable when we think about them, the appeal of getting to our weight goal in the shortest period of time is what is glaringly appealing. This initial appeal is not because we are weak. We are programmed to seek the easy way out, both in time and effort. Not because we are lazy, but because of nature's *fight or flight* instincts. Our natural instincts, unaddressed, make long-term success extremely difficult.

Successful people understand that they are never truly *stuck* nor limited by the short-term plan. They know that they can change the course of their lives by making choices outside their comfort zone, choosing the habits they want to form and slowly, but steadily, building the desires of their conscious thought.

Successful people are aware of the effort it takes to undo their old, set ways. They take that effort because they know that, with perseverance and persistence, they can create a whole new set of helpful, automatic responses to situations to build a whole new life.

THE WALL

Before we change our comfort zone, we need to break down the wall that surrounds it.

Think of our comfort zone as your personal mental kingdom and the *wall* as the fort around it. This *wall* protects our comfort zone from potential threats. In the last section, I mentioned how this *wall* is made up of all the limiting thoughts and statements that we tell ourselves. It uses our *mindset*, our automatic beliefs, against us when we try to change so that we feel *trapped* because of our own beliefs and attitudes.

On the other hand, the "happy" emotions we experience in our comfort zone also tempt us. We want the "happy" feeling over and over again; that comfort and assurance. Our mind will do whatever it takes to maintain these "happy" emotions to turn to what is comfortable. What do I mean?

Example: you have fully committed to a new, healthy eating and exercise plan. You are 100% certain that you will finally rid yourself of the excess weight that has held you back for so long. You dot every I and cross every T; you even see yourself thin, including your new wardrobe and all the increased energy you will have to be more active with your friends and family. You go full force into your new plan and even wake up early to tackle exercise.

Despite how it's all laid out, you soon grow tired. You find it extremely challenging to wake up so early, and those salads are less appetizing than the potlucks that everyone seems to be having since your new commitment. Your family is no help, even though they try, as they point out that *you're beautiful just the way you are* and should *just settle for your big bone stature that is a part of your genes.*

Although you still have high hopes of losing weight, you give into their theory and believe that perhaps your new regimen is too rigid. After all, gradual weight loss is better than rapid, right?

Your workouts become later and fewer; your meals become larger and less restrictive.

> Before you know it, you find yourself right back into familiar territory: added pounds, heightened frustration, revolving diets and very little progress to show for it.

In itself, this "*wall*" is not a bad thing. The mind built the *wall* around our comfort zone to keep us safe. The comfort zone is all the things we have learned, know and understand. Staying within its boundaries ensures that we are not at risk of the unknown; there we are protected and safe.

These are the beliefs, attitudes and options that we learned from our parents and grandparents – and other influential people close to us – because these were the people that protected us as children. They are also the beliefs that we learned from our friends, because these were the people who surrounded us and protected us from being alone. Thus, the comfort zone and the *wall* around it, are created to serve deep seated needs of safety and security, as well as love and affection that all humans share.

Hitting The Wall

But in trying to protect us, the *wall* also limits us in making and adapting to new lifestyle changes. How do we break the cycle of failure? Start by making new lifestyle choices, forcing you to leave your comfort zone. Understand that, in doing so, you will meet the *wall* of resistance.

Your weight set point is inside that comfort zone; your mind reacts against drastic weight loss by trying to dissuade you from breaking through the *wall*. This is why when you start a new eating or exercise routine, although you see some success with time, you eventually hit this *wall* and your mind starts to resist change. You begin to rationalize, or tell yourself "rational lies," and start to think of excuses for quitting this new routine, even though you may be following a healthy sustainable lifestyle.

You start having all kinds of internal conversations that focus on the negative aspects of your new changes and experiences. You are now hyper aware and super sensitive to any negative emotions or feedback received from your environment.

You hit this internal *wall* and BOOM, you start to ask yourself, "*Is this really worth it? Do I deserve to lose weight? Why do I need to lose weight anyway?*" You start to see things that *need* your attention more and you question the sense in starting a new regimen.

What will people think? You start to doubt your own motivations and abilities; you search out anything that will help you feel better again. For most, returning to old habits and lifestyle choices that are *comfortable or known,* is what predicts weight gain.

The *wall* that surrounds our comfort zone is built on fear, doubt and worry. Once you start to lose weight and try to leave your comfort zone, you will eventually hit this *wall*. Then you start to *fear* that you can't do it; you *doubt* the process you chose to do it; you doubt if you really can lose all the excess weight, and even if you do, you *worry* that you won't be able to maintain it. Even in this, the *wall* was designed for your benefit.

There is a reason the *wall* is built from our doubts, our fears and our worries. These are the emotions that are tasked with keeping us safe and ensuring that we do only the things that are proven to keep us functional. This is why, the moment we make a choice that takes us outside our comfort zone we start to question it, doubt it or worry about how or why we are even doing it. Even though we badly want change, our basal selves fear drastic change and try to avoid it at all cost. This creates a self-sabotaging lifestyle of thoughts and distractions that deter you from your goals.

Returning to the previous example, what emotions would you say pulled the dieter back into his or her comfort zone? What about the environment encouraged him or her to return back to old ways? We will explore this further in the next few paragraphs. First, I would like to make it personal:

> *What are some emotions that you feel may cause you to eat in unhelpful/helpful ways?*
>
> *What are some environmental factors in your life that cause you to eat in unhelpful/helpful ways?*

I want you to see how our comfort zone is surrounded by a *wall* that is made up of fear, doubt, and worry that can really lock us into this self-imposed prison. These emotions – fears, doubts, and worries, or our environment, is what feeds these emotions to work against any positive lifestyle change.

How Do We Break Through This Wall?

The only way to break through this *wall* is to make choices, and to take consistent actions, that are outside of your current comfort zone. Accept that change is *difficult;* there will be *"transitional costs."* These are the costs of being uncomfortable before you become comfortable with your new habits and lifestyle.

Transitional costs are the exercises you don't want to do but continue to do. This is the passing by of the unhealthy restaurants you used to visit on a regular basis. These are the negative, unsupportive emotions you feel when going through the process, and the environment you are around that doesn't support you or your new choices.

These are the costs you have to pay for your body and health to transition to who you want and deserve to be. The key is not to focus on the *"costs,"* but to focus on the benefits that you are getting from this new lifestyle. When I first started at the gym, I hated it. I used to set my alarm clock to go off at 6am, because I knew that if I didn't go to the gym first thing in the morning, then it wouldn't get done. But over time this became my routine and I developed the habit of going. Over time I started to feel better and it didn't seem so hard to get up any more to go. The *"costs"* kept decreasing while the benefits kept improving how I felt, how my body was changing, and the energy that I was feeling. I throughly believe that you don't pay the price for good health, you enjoy the benefits of good health.

In order to shift our comfort zone, we have to be aware of our discomfort and keep questioning it for some time. Successful people recognize that it takes time to break old habits and establish new ones. Thus, they ignore all the warnings when they break out of their comfort zones and keep persevering until they establish a new normal for themselves.

Remember, this *wall* is built from our worries, fears and doubts. So it is only natural that we will feel out of place, sometimes unhappy, uncomfortable and doubtful when we are breaking this *wall*. Fear of the new and unknown is natural; we should accept it as a sign that we are going in the right direction. But if we allow the fear to take over, it will automatically lead to doubt and then to worry, which will eventually halt our progress. You have to resolve to do all you can, resolve to do whatever it takes no matter of the costs and develop the *mindset* that the process will become easier the longer you stick with it.

The important thing to remember here is that, if we could build a comfort zone once, we can do it again. We just have to recognize and appreciate the effort that needs to be taken and keep practicing the good habits that will help us stay healthy. If we take action consistently, we will find ourselves in a new, healthier comfort zone that is built on healthy habits that are valuable to our well-being.

EMOTIONS

What you are eating is from what's eating you.

You may want to lose weight and get more fit. You exercise regularly, maybe even hit the gym consistently, but your diet is another story. You try your best but temptation often gets the best of you. On those days you think, "If only I could control my portions / choose healthy foods / stop overeating / stop binge eating /..." You know what needs to be avoided, but you can't seem to do what needs to be done although you try again and again and again...

You are not alone in your fight against unhealthy eating habits; for many of my clients, this is the norm. Even if you are trying to live a healthier lifestyle, you may find yourself constantly reaching for comfort foods or unhealthy snack foods as a source of comfort. Sometimes we do this without thought which sabotages our results. Then you may ask yourself, *why did I just do that?* When the mind must choose between deeply rooted emotions and logic, emotions almost always win.

Emotional Eating

Emotions have the ability to make us healthy or make us sick: they play a huge role in whether or not we achieve our goals. While our thoughts trigger emotions, it is our emotions that fuel our actions. Emotional eating, for example, is the act of using food to make ourselves feel better. Many of us eat to fulfill emotional needs rather than to fill the stomach. Unfortunately emotional eating doesn't fix problems; and it usually makes us feel worse in the long run.

Emotional "hunger" cannot be satisfied by food. We try to use food for comfort, but eating in unsupportive ways just triggers certain physiological reactions that temporarily provides relief as a distraction until the real problems resurface.

Caution: if you are an emotional eater, it is important to understand what emotional need is triggering your cravings. You could be using food to cope with something stressful, to distract yourself, to celebrate, to express happiness or to reduce the experience of being sad, anxious or upset.

Any emotion is capable of triggering food cravings if the association between emotion and food is strong enough. Most people do not discriminate when it comes to eating and emotions. Emotional eating is not a crime and it's perfectly acceptable to do it on occasions.

The real problem is when emotional eating becomes a major coping mechanism for the negative events in your life. Afterward, not only does the original emotional issue remain, but you are riddled with guilt for these actions.

2 Types Of Emotional Eating

There are two types of emotional eating that will stop you from achieving your desired lifestyle changes: emotional eating in reaction to daily triggers and emotional eating in reaction to your life change.

1. Daily Triggers

These are the daily thoughts and or experiences that cause emotional eating. A "*trigger*" is something that stimulates you to eat. Whether reaching for unhealthy snacks when you think about a past event/trauma or *needing* to turn to a comfort food because of something that happened at work, these emotional habits slowly sabotage your efforts to lose weight. You first need to understand "*why*" you are eating this way.

If you realize that you are not eating out of hunger, you have to figure out the triggers and habits that are driving you to eat. First it starts with awareness. You need to be aware of when you are eating in unhelpful/unhealthy ways, and once you have done that, you can then find effective ways to substitute unhealthy eating habits with other helpful actions.

Some of these daily triggers are external, and could be triggered by something as simple as watching a sad movie. According to food psychologist Brian Wansink, author of *Mindless Eating*, people watching sad movies eat 28 to 55 percent more food during that movie.

On the other hand, many people turn to sweets and cakes as a means of celebration when a happy event occurs. People will respond to different situations, both positive and negative, by eating. If you are doing this, you have to identify the more typical triggers for you and then find healthy alternatives for them.

For others, food is a way to cope with dramatic life incidents and the emotions accompanying these events. Through my experience, I am still amazed how many people still dwell over a past event – something that is now beyond their control, because it is in their past. Knowingly, or unknowingly, they eat to feel better about what happened long ago, which becomes a habit every time something triggers a memory.

Moving forward with a healthy eating plan and a new lifestyle means recognizing what is causing you to eat in unhelpful ways. Be prepared to come face to face with the issues, tragedies, and pain of your past.

Many of us associate being consistent with healthy food choices with being on a "diet." For some people, even hearing the word, "diet," causes feelings of failure, negativity, and anxiety. Many of my coaching clients say that "diet" to them means restriction, hunger, cravings, and memories of all the other times they failed on a weight loss plan. Understandably, this brings up feels of resentment that can derail your efforts before you get started.

Knowing It Will Happen

You have to control what you're eating or else it will get out of control.

Sometimes eating out of emotion will happen. But it's when emotional eating becomes a major coping mechanism that you have an issue of epic concern.

Our food choices contribute to our overall health and weight. So, when you eat to control your moods as a response to everyday irritations, situations and concerns, you are setting yourself up for failure without even realizing it.

Just being aware of these little triggers can be enough to get back on track. You have to be vigilant about *what* and *why* you are eating. Once you realize that you are not eating out of hunger, you have to figure out the specific triggers and habits that drive you to eat.

Meeting The Problem

Identify which emotions are triggering unhealthy eating. When you know what prompts you to reach for these foods, it is easier to challenge yourself, stop or modify the action and create solutions. We all have an "*emotional home*" that we go to. Happy people find a way to be happy. Stressful people find ways to stress. It's identifying which of these emotions that contently come up that are causing you to eat in unhelpful ways.

One of the best ways to find these is to keep a meal log or journal and write down what you eat – when you eat, how much and how you are feeling when you eat. If you suspect serious emotional eating, make a note of how you felt before you chose your meal or snack and how you felt after you ate it.

I know this may sound like a lot to do, but it only takes a couple minutes each day to write down these details. Over just a few weeks, your log or journal will provide you with incredible data that you can use to help yourself moving forward. As the days pass, you may see patterns emerge that reveal the connections between your moods and your food choices and preferences.

Once you have this data, you should start tracking the trends that appear in your food choices and moods. It can be stressful, and maybe even embarrassing at times, but you have to figure out why you are eating what you are eating. It's important to understand which internal experiences are causing you to eat in unhelpful ways.

All eating starts with a trigger. This trigger – which is a situation that stimulates you to eat – could be physiological hunger, a mental rule or norm, an environmental or social cue to eat (like meeting up with a friend), or an emotional trigger.

Physiological hunger means that your body needs sustenance. An environmental trigger could be something you saw on TV that prompts a craving or a social cue to eat as a means of fitting in with people. Personal rules or norms are a matter of habit – for example, eating lunch at 1 pm regardless of whether you are hungry.

All of these are more or less within our control; we can modify our decision to eat, our food and portion choices or whether/how we respond to these cues. But, most importantly, we need to identify and understand our emotional cues to eating. Once we understand our emotional triggers and respond to them, controlling the other factors will become a lot easier.

One way to do this is to take stock of what foods you are reaching for to fill emotional needs. Looking at what you're eating could be a way of looking at what emotional needs you are trying to remedy. According to Psychoanalyst Dr. Nina Savelle-Rocklin, who specializes in weight, body image, and disordered eating, when you do not know what is going on internally, you should take a good look at what your mind is craving, food wise. Dr. Nina suggests that identifying trends in the kind of comfort foods you prefer when you are under emotional duress, can pinpoint emotional issues you may be experiencing without even being aware. She suggests four categories:

Ice cream, frozen yogurt and pudding – Soothing, creamy textures are preferred when we long for comfort. People who choose these foods often are likely to feel a void in their life.

Candy and sweets – We turn to sweet foods when we feel that there is not enough sweetness, kindness, love, and attention in our lives. We use these foods to fill the need to be cared for or to make up for an unfulfilling relationship.

Bread, bagels, cake and muffins – These bulky, filling foods are preferred by people when they feel lonely, empty, or deprived. People tend to turn towards these foods when they feel like they can't cope with their life events or when they feel that they are misunderstood by others.

Potato chips, pretzels, crackers and other savoury snacks – Crunchy foods and snacks are preferred when we are in a bad mood of some sort. It could be anger, frustration, annoyance, or irritation that makes us reach for that bag of chips.

Reminder: Before we change any of our habits, we need to be aware of what we are eating and why. Not just for any one day but on a weekly and even monthly basis. Keeping a meal log or journal will help you identify these eating patterns in your life. This will help you understand what the problems are and to decide what you can do to change the situation that triggers unhelpful eating behaviours.

Knowing why you partake in emotional eating is only the first step. Sometimes just the awareness helps in controlling some of your cravings (or at least portion sizes). But often it is not enough. You have to look for solutions.

2. Eating From Change

We also can turn to emotional eating when we experience change – even a change we like. This is because comfort foods are things we have been used to since childhood. Creating a new healthy lifestyle that doesn't include or alters comfort food, for most people, is a huge change. So *thinking* of all the changes you may have to make in your life and what you will have to go through, can also trigger undesirable eating.

How often has the following happened to you?

> You feel like you've made some progress towards controlling your emotional eating: you've found a good nutrition plan and exercise routine; you've bought an organizer to put everything in and make your regimen official; and you've bought new Tupperware to store all the healthy meals you plan to prepare. And you are still missing the mark; you still can't get started.
>
> You are motivated and confident about your choices. Even though you've found ways to keep yourself inspired, you

still find yourself hesitant about starting. You worry that you will take two steps forward only to take three steps back.

What is the problem in the above scenario? Your *mindset*. The moment you start working towards a goal that takes you out of your comfort zone, non-supportive self-talk starts and derails your progress. Your *mindset* – which influences your emotions and your habits – keeps you from fully committing to the new regimen.

Although you started out positive, your mental chatter soon changes into negative, stressful thoughts that only sabotage you further by making you crave more comfort foods. And so you eat in a quest to feel better.

The negative thoughts and emotions that send you scrambling for comfort foods, draws on your subconscious body image from environmental cues that question your new choices. You are now afraid to move forward and the fear paralyzes your progress.

The truth is, at an unconscious level, you are afraid of changing, afraid of eating different, afraid of losing weight and afraid of getting healthier. This fear of change stops your progress and keeps you from breaking out of your comfort zone and sustaining your efforts.

The Fear Of Life Changes

Fear may seem like an unjustified emotion in this situation of creating a healthy life change, but when you think of it, fear is perfectly logical. Everyone has many fears, small and large, that guide their daily actions. But fear, out of control, can paralyze us and keep us from taking constructive action in the direction of our goals.

From the thousands of clients I have coached, I have found three common types of fear that hinder us from attaining our healthy lifestyle goals:

1. The fear of change itself

> We worry that somehow the changes that we are making may affect our core self. We worry that *we might lose something we like about ourselves*. We fear that we won't be the same person and that we may not like the person we become.
>
> It is important to face this fear because the concern is an important one. We have to work through the idea that, even though we are adopting new behaviours and habits, our core personality and values will not change. One way to work through this fear is to identify things about ourselves that we want to keep constant and make note of this. We then have to ensure that our new choices and actions are consistent with these aspects. When we

understand this, we are ready to go ahead and stay the same person, while gaining a more fit and healthier body.

2. *The fear of the process*

Doing anything new is hard. We have to evaluate the demands of the new activity, make time and space for the new habits and decide what we have to give up or modify.

That fearful mind always ask *what if* questions: *What if it doesn't work? What if I can't do it? What if it's too hard?*

These are the challenges to change that we have to understand and work through. For most things that hold us back, there are alternatives and options that will work just as effectively. It is up to us to find and choose the ones that are best suited for us. Welcome the challenges and know that, with every challenge you face in your journey, there is a chance to learn about yourself and the situation. Every learning experience will bring you closer to where you want to be.

3. *The fear of the outcome*

Are you afraid of success especially when it comes to weight loss and healthy living? You may think, no way. But deep down you may think people will treat you differently if you change. We can also be afraid of success because of the fear that we will not be able to maintain it. This is particularly true for someone who has lost and regained weight before.

We can also be afraid of failure in regards to how we will be judged if we fail. If we're honest with ourselves, most of us spend a lot of time worried about what others think about us, including those in our immediate circle. Unchecked, this worry soon turns into fear. Often those who struggle with their weight, are afraid of how friends and others will react to their new lifestyle and future weight loss. They fear that others won't like or accept their changes.

Again, we need to find ways to explain our choices to friends and family so that they are supportive. It is important to help ourselves understand that *any results* are better than none. Remember, sustained results are simply a matter of changing our comfort zone over time which begins with a change in your *mindset*.

Keeping a journal or making notes in your food log can help you identify these emotions and fears and you may begin to understand the specific issues that can sabotage your success. If you have a thought that guides your food choices, write it down. Initially, just focus on gaining an awareness of these fears. Once you know what emotions hold you back, you can start to address this.

Remember, these are your emotions and thoughts; with the right guidance, you can respond to them effectively. You are IN

CONTROL: you CAN replace negative, sabotaging thoughts with more helpful ones, and address the emotions and needs that drive you to eat. You CAN activate the emotions that fuel healthy eating habits for the transformation you seek.

Making The Change

> *First comes awareness, then create an understanding, so you can find solutions.*

It's really important for you to *identify the emotions* that are causing you to eat in unhelpful ways so that you have the *power to change* the <u>meaning you give</u> to those emotions. This involves changing the response you give when these emotions are triggered. *Remember, using your meal log or journal is a great way to retrieve this data about yourself.*

One thing to remember is that *you choose* the thoughts you entertain, the emotions you feel and the actions you take. The emphasis is not so much the emotion you feel but the meaning you attach to that emotion. Choose meanings to emotions that empower you instead of those that disempower you. Choose meanings to emotions that are constructive versus destructive.

> For example, your feel stressed out, which triggers the emotion of helplessness. You are

worried, anxious, and you just want to make the world go away. You need a moment to breathe and relax. You decide to take some much needed time and relax at home, with your favourite meal, including wine, snack foods, and a decadent dessert. Sure, you're trying to lose weight and get healthier, but you need to relax and you can always work harder in the gym to make up for this one night of stress relief. Sound familiar?

The action you took to soothe yourself was overeating. Someone else's solution to a high stress period might have been going outside for a walk or having a hot bubble bath. Truthfully, you could have chosen the latter to produce the type of relief you needed. Choosing your responses to emotions, after assigning the appropriate meaning to them, will empower you instead of controlling you. You can choose to change a destructive situation into a constructive one. It is your choice.

When we indulge in destructive eating without advance planning or preparation, we feel guilt. These feelings of guilt are good: they alert us that change is needed.

Listen to the message your body is giving you. If you feel guilty, you have obviously taken an action that is counterproductive or not aligned to the results you seek. You are working against your goals and you need to get back into alignment instead of continuing on the path. Equate this as making the wrong turn: don't continue to drive the wrong way; turnaround and get back on course.

Maybe you ate too much of something that wasn't healthy for you; or "gave into" foods that you didn't really want to eat. In either case, your emotions are telling you that your choice of action was not in line with your goals. Use these feelings as a signal to make a change.

You can't change what has already occurred but you can learn from it and plan for the next time you find yourself in a similar situation. Perhaps the plan will involve eating less, eating something different or avoiding the situation completely.

When you have a plan, you will be ready to face the situation and respond to it in a different, more helpful manner. This means that you are less likely to feel guilty which, in and of itself, is the perfect reward for your changed behaviour.

For example, I never feel guilty about eating something because, if I *choose* to eat off plan, I have chosen to do so in advance. (Notice I said that I *choose* to do so and I planned for it *in advance*.) If I choose to eat something that I do not eat regularly, planning to do so, helps me to structure my meals and exercise plan the next day to get right back on track.

Let's say I ate something that I didn't plan for in advance, as sometimes life circumstances get in the way. I learn from it, and how to compensate for it, because now I am in a better position to pre-plan the next time this occurs. Sometimes things happen that you feel are out of your control. Be in control by learning from the experience and how to plan for it the next time it happens. (Because typically it does.)

Responding to the emotional appeal of food is all about how you feel about the past, how you feel about your present and how you feel about your future. You have to fight emotion with emotion – we will talk more about how to do this in the section on motivation.

ENVIRONMENT

If you don't program your environment, it will program you.

How Our Environment Affects Eating

The environment we live in plays a major role in the way we live. Specifically, in the context of health, it shapes our food choices, determines how sedentary or active we are and also influences our lifestyle choices from the options made available to us.

While our genes play a role in our ability to lose weight, our environment is what is mostly responsible for the specific everyday choices that we tend to make. It is not your genetics but your lifestyle that will make you overweight.

I agree that some people can lose weight faster than others based on their genetics, and yes, it's harder to lose weight for some versus others. But, if you are overweight, you can lose it.

Your environment trumps your genetics any day of the week when it comes to getting rid of weight and achieving healthy lifestyle goals.

Our environment can be rather unsupportive of a healthy lifestyle. For most of us, our work involves sitting in one place. Technology is rapidly making most forms of physical exertion or exercise redundant. Although most of these options are aimed at making our life easier, they can be counterproductive to our health goals.

We have access to more highly processed foods that are energy dense and nutritionally void or chemically dense compared to fresh, nutritious meals. Highly processed foods are often readily available, easily prepared and cheaper than nutritious, fresh food items. Unhealthy foods are offered in so many restaurants and at every corner. Particularly, a lot of the fast food chains serve some of the most processed, energy dense food, and thanks to effective marketing campaigns, they have widespread appeal.

Fast food chains lure people in with coupons sent through the mail as well as flyers and discounts. All marketing is geared to entice you to drive through and purchase their food offerings. Given the demands of most jobs, families and individuals seem to think that they have very little time to prepare home-cooked meals and are drawn to these foods. It's no wonder that about two-thirds of North Americans are overweight or obese.

The media is also a contributing factor to the obesity epidemic. We are flooded with commercials advertising processed, rich, and unhealthy food choices. So many of my clients tell me that they are motivated to consume unhealthy night time snacks because of a food commercial they saw. Children are also captivated by the snacks advertised and want to choose them over healthy snack options.

According to Dr. Brian Wansink, author of Mindless Eating, people who watch food related programming food are 11 pounds heavier, specifically those who cook a lot. This fact may be caused by the constant enticement to try energy dense recipes instead of simple, healthy ones. Even when people actively try to resist these messages, the subliminal messages remain in our minds and slowly influence our food choices.

The mixed messages we receive about food and health can leave many people vulnerable to eating disorders. The social pressure to be thin can add to the shame and fear that binge eaters feel, and these emotions further fuel unhealthy eating.

For many, our work and home spaces are not safe either. The office lunch room, break room, or cafeteria is constantly filled with tempting treats and snacks for the busy worker. Many people keep candy jars at their desks or in common areas; the perfect trap to having a sugar rush in the afternoon or regular sweet treats. Friends and co-workers will also offer each other treats or snacks, increasing the temptation even more.

For many of us, our home can make or break our healthy eating. If we keep our homes stocked with fresh, healthy foods, we are more likely to eat them. But often, people find excuses for why they have "very little time to cook" and turn to fast food, processed meals and unhealthy snacks at the end of a very busy day.

The #1 Environmental Factor – Other People

There are so many environmental factors that influence how we follow through with our health goals. But the #1 factor is who we surround ourselves with. Our friends, family, colleagues and other significant individuals play a vital role in how we look at food, what choices we make, what exercise we do or don't do, and how healthy we stay. Often we don't realize how easy it is for others to influence our food and fitness choices.

In his book "Connected," Dr. Nicholas Christatcis explains how our social circles influence our weight. The more overweight your friends are, the more likely you are to be overweight. Based on hard data and relationship analysis, he found that the impact of others weight on our own is far reaching – as far as the fourth degree of separation. According to Dr. Christatcis, if your friends are obese your chances of being obese increases by 45%; if your friend's friend is obese, your risk of obesity is 25% higher. Even the friend of a friend of a friend can influence our weight by increasing your risk of obesity by 10%, and this is likely to be someone you don't even know.

According to Dr. Christatcis, only when you get to your friend's- friend's- friend's - friends is there no correlation between that person's body size and your chances of obesity.

The infectious nature of the health of our social circle is because of the food and inactive habits that people pass to one another. When we socialize, we are influenced by each other's food choices and we tend to order and consume food that helps us bond or to fit in with the people we are with.

Habits and preferences that we pick up from one friend can then be passed onto another, thus evoking the contagious nature of unhealthy food habits. It is no wonder then that Dr. Nicholas Christatcis also found that when a friend of yours gains weight, the chances that you will gain weight during the same time period is nearly 57%.

Sometimes it's not what you know, it's who you know.

You and your choices are a reflection of your closest circle. The top 5 people you spend time with will slowly and surely influence your decisions, sometimes unknowingly. *What do they like to eat? How much and when do they eat? Do they exercise and how often?* All these factors play a role in influencing your personal choices as well.

Food Buddies VS. Food Bullies

Once you decide that you want to make a lifestyle change, you will find that the people around you are divided into two groups:

Supportive, nourishing people – these are the people who bring out the best in you. They take the effort to support your choices and inspire and motivate you to stay on your new path.

They hold you up, not hold you back. When you feel like slipping up, they keep you accountable and stop you from going back. When you meet someone who is supportive of your choices and decisions, you need to nurture that relationship. These people will become your support system throughout your journey and they will help you see the positive side on days when you cannot. Everyone hits hurdles in their journey but supportive people help you see your way past those hurdles.

Negative, toxic people – these are the people that you should be worried about. They are critical and create self-doubt for you by questioning your motives and your abilities. They are always telling you what you can't do and what problems you will face. They actually contribute to your failure, as they are demotivating and exhausting to be around. When someone acts like this, find a way to distance yourself from them.

Try to shield your new habits from them, as they are likely to hold you back. Most people never achieve their goals in life because they are surrounded by too many toxic, negative, energy draining people. Negative people teach us how NOT to think. They keep focusing on the failures, on the problems and on the conflicts. Look at them as an example of what kind of thoughts can hold a person back and strive to not practice the same.

You have to know who you can count on, and who you should count out.

Sometimes I have clients who have a supportive environment, for a while, when they start their new lifestyle. Then, suddenly, they start experiencing resistance from the people around them. Family or friends who were supportive in the beginning, start becoming critical as they get closer and closer to their goals.

This can be very disheartening to deal with and many people lose the motivation to continue with their efforts afterwards. But why do people who were your cheerleaders suddenly turn against your success?

As mentioned earlier, the reason why it is so hard for you to change is the same reason it is so hard for the people around us to adapt to change. *People want change but they resist being changed.* As they see you making these changes and losing weight while increasing your health, they may feel obligated to do the same so as not to be left behind. This sense of urgency takes them out of their own comfort zone and they immediately respond by establishing a *wall* of defence. Often, without consciously planning to do so, they now try to hold you back to where you started which releases their self-imposed pressure.

These people now can become food bullies or food pushers and end up sabotaging your results and goals. They will say things like, "Just try one; I made it for you" or "Oh have this, just this once; it's the weekend." My mother is a prime example of this. She can be a food bully. You have to be careful when she is serving you food. Don't get me wrong, she's a great cook but she is allergic to empty plates.

My mother fills up your plate until nothing else can possibly fit on it. If you can possibly finish what's on your plate, she will constantly refill it if you are not looking. You have to keep an eye on your plate at all times if you are over to her house for a meal. (*She will refill that plate faster than a speeding bullet.*)

I now politely ask to serve my own food when I go for a visit. If you have someone like this around you, you need to pay special attention so that they don't derail your progress. (Please do so without being rude to them. Remember, these people love you but are victims of their own conditioning.) Be kind, but firm with them and do not let them influence you with unhelpful behaviours.

I had a client that used to see me every Thursday night. She was a retired teacher and had about 140 lbs. to lose to get to a healthy weight. She had tried everything to lose weight before but nothing seemed to work for her long term.

I met her at her heaviest and she was ready to take the effort needed to change her life around. She did great. She started to eat healthy and to become more active. Her mother, who lived about five hours away from her, used to call her every Thursday night to check on her after she left my clinic.

Her mother was really supportive in the beginning and would encourage her. But after my client lost her first 30 lbs., she found that her mother's calls started to change. They went from encouraging to discouraging, so much so that, at the end of the conversation, she would feel demotivated and the impact of our sessions would be wiped out.

Even though my client was eating healthier than ever and losing about 1 – 2 lbs. a week, her mother was skeptical. She would say things like, "*You are losing the weight too fast; you are not going to maintain it*" or "*This isn't healthy; this won't last.*" My client started to dread her mother's calls because she knew that she was doing the right thing and becoming healthier with her rightful choice.

Thankfully, my client found the strength to ignore the messages she was receiving. She knew that the regimen was working for her and she saw the results. She was eliminating all the excess weight she had carried all her life. Even though she stayed in touch with her mother every Thursday, she told me that she "*would hear everything her mother was saying to her but had to stop listening to her when it came to her weight and lifestyle.*" She further added:

"That this is what happens every time that I start to live a healthier lifestyle and try to lose this weight. My mother is always at me to lose the weight, but when I start losing the weight, my mother always talks me out of it, even though I'm at such an unhealthy weight."

I am happy to report that my client kept losing the weight and meeting all goals until she hit her target. She says that the only reason she was able to resist the criticism was that she was aware and alert this time, because she knew what was happening and would not let it happen again, so she tuned it out.

It is better to be disliked by others than to be disliked by yourself.

The take away from this story is that the people around you don't always know what's best FOR YOU. They may be persuasive but you need to decide what messages to take and which ones to ignore. Rather than trying to change the negative people, you need to focus within and use the lessons you have learned, negative and positive, to improve your outcome.

People may often doubt you because they have seen you fail before. Show them, through your continued efforts, that you are serious this time. Those who love you will eventually understand how hard you have worked and will come around. This may take some time but the best way to convince them is through consistent action. *You have to win over them to win them over.*

Relationships exert a powerful influence on our goal achievements in a number of ways. Sometimes family members and friends are supportive in voice but not by actions. They want you to continue to eat the same things that they have always eaten. They don't want to tempt you purposely, but they don't realize how hard of a time you are having.

During such times, have a conversation with them and explain your experiences, in the hope of finding a middle ground. A middle ground where your goals don't have to force them to take steps they don't want to and their food choices do not conflict with your goals. Unfortunately, a lot of people give up before they try to talk things through with the people closest to them.

Role Models

A lot of people expect other people to change in order to make them happy, healthy and fit. It doesn't work that way. The change has to come from you.

But one of the best ways to start improving your health is to be around people that are already living a healthy lifestyle. Maybe they have demonstrated habits of success, like living a healthy lifestyle where they have lost weight and kept it off. If no one around you is currently doing this, don't expect them to change; seek out those who are. Get around people that are demonstrating the results you want to achieve.

How? Join a workout class, walk group, a healthy cooking class, or you may want to hire a food coach and or personal trainer. The more you are around these people, the more they will influence your behaviour. Successful people look at other successful people as a means to motivate themselves. They see other successful people as models to learn from.

For those of you that are surrounded by toxic people when it comes to your lifestyle goals, never let anyone tell you what you *cannot do*, especially if they have not done it themselves. I find this all the time in the health and wellness industry, especially concerning weight loss. Absolutely refuse to spend another day living the way someone else wants you to live. Someone else does not know what is possible for you, but they can influence your motivation.

Find people who will help you gain success by being an example. When you have reached your goal, you can also be the same support to someone else who is struggling as you are now. Often we cannot rid our lives completely of the negative toxic people, especially if they are part of our closest family and friends. What we can do though, is add more people to our circle that will help us stay on track.

It can be a great idea to hire a coach or find a mentor. These people understand your journey and know what will help you reach your goals. They provide both an example and a push for the days when you can't visualize yourself reaching your goal. They help you find the strength to push through the fatigue, discouragement and confusion. They help you to see alternatives that you are unable to see. Use yourself and their personal experiences to help you decide between choices when you are confused. And, as your circle expands to include these positive influences, the doubters in your life can also be inspired to see your goals in a positive light.

Another option is to create a buddy system with someone else that is trying to achieve the same goals. When someone you trust – like a friend, family member, or colleague – has the same goals as you, it can help to team up so both parties stay focused and accountable throughout the process.

Although coaches and professionals play a vital role in helping you make decisions and monitoring your progress, a "health-buddy" can be the difference between success and failure. He or she makes it easier to avoid certain foods and to exercise regularly because you have an accountability partner. Similarly, they receive the same encouragement, support and feedback from you that you receive from them. This keeps both people on track.

Another valuable aspect of the buddy system is that you can evaluate your different experiences. With this type of support relationship, you both gain invaluable knowledge to further your success.

Creating An Environment Of Support

Everyone has a certain number of supportive and non-supportive people around them. Find out who can form your support system and spend more time with them. If there are people around you who you share different goals with, interact with them all.

If you are someone who gets bored of exercising alone, consider joining a class or an organized group. For a number of people, the social network they form around their habits and activities are a vital motivator. If you are one of these people, use the social aspect of food and exercise groups to help keep you motivated, connected and on track.

For others, professionals can be a great source of motivation, information and support. If this works for you, consider hiring a coach, nutritionist, dietitian, or personal trainer or see your doctor, to help you work through the difficult parts.

A "coach" doesn't necessarily have to be a clinician or professional; he or she can be someone who understands your journey and who you trust. Others gain from using affirmations or from meditation that helps them modify their personal thoughts. All these are tools for success and each person should try to find the tools that best enable them to stay active, eat right and stay focused on their goals.

People who have struggled for a long time often do best when they combine many different support systems. They may even form a "team" – perhaps some combination of doctors, coaches, nutritionists, exercise classes, support groups or a buddy.

CHANGE

Throughout the first part of this book, we have discussed how the different elements of your life – the people you surround yourself with, your upbringing and your life circumstances – all play a role in what you weigh, how much or how little exercise you do and what you choose to eat. They all have had an influence in creating your *mindset* and are layers of the *wall* you've built around your comfort zone.

Armed with this awareness, let's examine the basic framework of change that is required for you to apply in order to change your *mindset*, break the *wall* and re-establish a comfort zone that encourages healthier habits.

You know by now that the first step to lasting change in your weight and health is to change your *mindset*. But how?

> ***It starts with an idea – the idea that you are going to change your life.***

You have to articulate this to yourself, over and over again, until you truly believe it. You need to make this idea powerful. How? By adding emotion to it. I will give you a more detailed guide to doing this in the next part of this book. But for the moment, make a commitment to yourself that you will take the necessary steps to change your life and take charge of your health.

You are now aware that your *mindset* is the reason you entertain the thoughts you think and the actions you take. You have to change your thinking if you want to change your life. If you could form a set of automatic habits and responses once, you can do it again. You can consciously choose and control your thoughts; what you think and believe is what you will have.

There will always be negative, non-supportive thoughts but you get to choose to focus on the positive, constructive, and supportive ones. Although it takes time and practice, the non-supportive thoughts will start to die from malnutrition, and the positive, more constructive ones that you nourish, will produce the type of actions that allow you to achieve your goals.

The game is long term change – each day, you will have to remind yourself of your new choices, new goals and new actions until they become second nature (they will with time). Someone once told me that, "The best diet is the one that you don't know you're on." That is when you will know that you are truly changing your lifestyle and your life.

Until then, learn from your successes and use failures as a lesson in finding more effective ways to get the results you desire. This book will serve as your blueprint to creating the *mindset* needed for successful change and give you the action steps needed to obtain the long-term results you desire.

First You Have To Change The Way

If you change the way you look at food, you will change the way you look.

Most people view food as a means to survive, not to thrive. If you start to look at food as a tool that helps you thrive and become a better, healthier version of yourself, you will find yourself reaching less for foods that hinder your success and body/health goals. If you focus on being a healthier person overall, you will find that your new food choices and exercises make you feel better. They give you better health, more energy, a better immune system and improved digestion.

Look at food as the fuel for your actions versus the dead weight that brings you down. Remember, if you are trying to lose weight, a healthy weight is a by-product of healthy eating. You will achieve a healthy weight and optimum health by living a healthy lifestyle. See food as your medicine. Living a healthy lifestyle is also your preventive medicine for the now and the future.

Another way to change your *mindset* is by your actions. You have to keep on practicing the new healthy behaviours until they become habits and the new thoughts until they become automatic. Repetition – of your thoughts and actions – is the only way to ensure enduring and efficient change over time.

How is your *mindset* developed? Through repetition of information and action. How do you change your *mindset*? Through repetition of information and action. A change in your *mindset* equals a change in your life.

Remember, the choices you make for the new you will be outside of your comfort zone. These choices are that of the person you want to become – the healthier, perhaps slimmer, you. It will take great mental effort, followed by practice, to normalize these new thoughts and habits. But, if you are truly ready this time, it will happen for you, and this book will help you accomplish it.

To break out of your comfort zone, you have to make choices and take actions outside of the norm. Start by taking new daily actions where you are moving towards your goals. Like an elastic band, you have to stretch yourself but not to the point where you snap.

You have to make goals that are difficult enough to stretch you out of your comfort zone but are achievable. For example, you are not going to run a marathon next week if you never have before. Take baby steps. Start by talking to a runner or trainer or buy a book or DVD on how to run. Start walking or jogging a couple times a week and continue from there.

A lot of times people burn themselves out creating a new lifestyle that is too much, too soon. They stretch themselves too far, too quickly and they snap. Get into the Elastic Zone; when motivation is high, stretch further. When motivation is low, stretch less but keep moving forward and keep stretching yourself.

The most effective way to do this is to take daily actions that slowly take you away from your current lifestyle and towards your new, healthier one. Remember that each new goal should challenge you, but should also be practical and possible.

Also, remember to pay attention to your emotional needs. There will be days when you are highly motivated – use these opportunities to stretch your limits by adding in new challenges. But you will also have days when you are feeling so low that you don't feel like pushing yourself at all. On such days, do the minimum to move you forward, that you set for yourself, but then cut yourself some slack.

In the journey to forming a new *mindset* and thinking a new way – feeling different emotions and changing your daily behaviours – you are going to feel uncomfortable. This has to be expected for you or anyone going through the process of a lifestyle change. Anytime you leave your current comfort zone, you have to expect to be uncomfortable. Unfortunately there are *"transitional costs."*

Remember, transitional costs are the costs you pay for your body going through this transition. Some of the costs include emotional downs, discomfort in certain situations, and maybe even losing people who will not follow the "new you." But do not focus on the costs; focus on the benefits you are getting from this healthier lifestyle. Focusing on the costs, which most people do, will halt your success. Remind yourself that the little time of initial discomfort, will help you reap long-term benefits for the rest of your life.

Meanings Of Emotions

While it's not the easiest thing to do, you can change the meaning you give to your emotions. This is vital because certain emotions attached to certain meanings can result in destructive actions.

You can learn to substitute and change destructive emotions with constructive ones, by first changing your thoughts. While it takes time to identify sabotaging thoughts and substitute them with helpful ones, this habit will yield you rewards in all aspects of your life, not just health.

For example, thinking of something you are grateful for when you are frustrated, will help you feel more in control and will improve your mood. Gratefulness is one of the strongest emotions you can feel.

When you focus on the positive alternative to a negative thought and take action on it, this is where personal power comes from. This is powerful and we will talk more about this in part 2 of this book.

If you find your negative self-talk overwhelming, start listening to motivational, inspirational messages. Also you can, *and should*, re-read this book to reaffirm your new path whenever you feel like you are headed in the wrong direction.

Environment And Food

The things around you can change the course of your lifestyle. Pay attention to the little things that surround you in life. *What are you watching? What are you listening to? What foods do you have in your home? What's in your kitchen at home and at work? What foods are on the table? What are you bringing to work every day to eat? Who are the people you are influenced by?* All of these affect what you are thinking about, what you are eating and what activities you are doing on a daily basis.

Be diligent about ridding your environment of things that can – *and will* – derail you. Add things to your environment that will help you stay on track. Find out what helps you and use that to keep you motivated.

We now know how our choices are affected by our past conditioning and environment (including childhood). We know how difficult it is to break away from long-term habits.

Understand that it is unfair to make yourself do too much too soon. (I know, no one typically tells you that, but that is what is causing you to fail). Pay special attention to this because people tend to sabotage themselves when they push too hard, too fast, and for too long.

Many people who start new routines, even with good intentions, slip back into old habits in a few weeks when they discover that their new routine was not "livable." Doing things one step at a time, and finding ways to incorporate new daily actions into your lifestyle, may take a little longer to see the results but the results will be more lasting.

Understanding your likes and dislikes may be the difference between success and failure. *What are some healthy foods you want to incorporate into your diet? What can you do right now to be more active? What healthy foods do you already like to eat? What are some you haven't tried before that you are willing to try? What activity or exercise do you like to do? What are some you haven't tried before that you would like or willing to try?*

Our mind and body give us valuable feedback when we are making changes. It is necessary to take this feedback in consideration when making long-term choices. After all, you are more likely to continue doing something that makes sense to you than something that does not. And when you find the options that work for you, you will find yourself more motivated and feeling great about becoming healthier.

For example, you know that feeling you get after a big Thanksgiving or holiday dinner? Sure, at first you enjoyed all the many tasty selections and decadent desserts. After all, this only happens once a year; why not indulge? As you sit around the table with those you hold dear, you unbuckle your belt and eat like there is no tomorrow!

Well, you know what happens soon after. You're stuffed beyond capacity, you're tired and all you want to do is go to bed. You may experience indigestion and have to take antacids or fizzy tablets to feel better. Your *food coma* often extends to the morning after and you feel sluggish and tired. You are suffering from a *food hangover*. What seemed like a fun filled, justifiable experience actually is one of the best lessons of how our body responds based on what we put in it.

People And Their Expectations

Other people around you may also unwittingly sabotage you, sometimes without even knowing they are doing so. Some don't mean to and some do, but remember that when you change your behaviours, you are causing change for them too. And since they didn't plan this change, it may be met with resistance.

Remember that they are just responding to the changes in their lives versus trying to purposely make you unhealthy. Do not demand that they have to live your lifestyle or that they practice the same plan. In time, they will adjust to accommodate your new choices. The idea here is to be the model of success; *win over them to win them over*. Win this battle of life change, and they may even get inspired to practice more healthy habits themselves. Be consistent with your new choices and actions and let them do it at their own pace.

If we know that the people around us influence our choices, let's understand how to respond to these people. Find out which people in your environment are supportive of you and which are toxic to your efforts. Remember that resistance to change is to be expected from those whom it affects but you need to be ready with responses to these situations. Instead of worrying about what they think or how they feel, explain your stand, come to an understanding, make some compromises with them and then do your thing. Hopefully when they see the positive changes you are making, they will be inspired to support you and to incorporate some of your habits. If not, you have your health and well-being to be concerned with. You cannot change people and how they will react, but you can change your responses to them.

Some people are likely to take objection to your change and may insist that you eat like you used to or not exercise. Particularly with family members and friends, they often use food for almost every occasion, event or circumstance. Your new healthy lifestyle will trigger a lot of demands and questions.

You may feel guilty about your change with them, but remember that this is something you must do for *yourself*. At the same time, recognize that they are not trying to hurt you. Their ideas about food were also conditioned and derived from different times and circumstances, many of these habits have been passed down from generations. Explain to your loved ones that you are making choices that are in line with the rest of your life and the quality of it.

Spouses and partners can be tricky to deal with when making major lifestyle changes. This is because when only one partner makes a lifestyle choice, there can be a mismatch that makes both partners uncomfortable. If you are making the choice to change things, sit your partner down and discuss why you are making the changes you have decided to make. Discuss how each of you feel – about food, meals, snacks, portions, health, fitness, and exercise – and how these feelings feed your individual and joint habits.

Knowing the reasons for each other's decisions and preferences can help in accepting differences where they exist. Be ready to make adjustments for your partner to lead the life they want to at the moment. But, at the same time, the plan of action that you come up with should be something that works for you as a couple, not just as individuals. You will be able to find common ground when you search for it and ask for it. Take that as a starting point to get used to each other's choices. Also be ready for an adjustment phase while this happens.

For example, you have decided that it is time for you and your partner to eat healthy and exercise so you can live a better quality of life and set healthy habits for your children. You devise a healthy regimen that includes early morning walks, taking your lunch to work, and preparing all your meals at home, except for family dinner out once a week.

You're fully committed, but after a few days, your partner is not as enthusiastic or willing. He or she doesn't want to get up so early in the morning or eat packed lunches every day. He or she plans to compensate by working out during their lunch hour and eating a larger breakfast and prepared snacks to hold them until dinner time.

You are upset because you feel it would be easier if you both followed the same routine. This is the wrong approach. Count your blessings that your partner still wants to commit to a healthy lifestyle, just not your way. That actually is preferred; in order to make a lifestyle change, you must know how to balance your choices, despite your surroundings and circumstances. Encourage your partner's efforts while following a different path. Look for similarities where you can both participate and share your progress, successes and revised plans for obstacles and challenges.

Surround Yourself With The Right People

Remember: we adjust to the standards of the people we are around the most. What are their views on living a healthy lifestyle, on nutrition or physical activity? If you truly want to make lasting changes in your life, it is important to be around people with the same *mindset* that you want to have. If you are not motivated, get around motivated people. If you are not living the healthy lifestyle that you want to live, find a way to spend time with people who are living it. This is a sure fire way to start changing your *mindset* and your results.

Where possible, try to interact more with people who share your views on health, lifestyle, and nutrition; less with those who do not. Particularly, when you are in the initial stages of your lifestyle change, it is essential to surround yourself with supporters and similar minded people, as these people will motivate and inspire you to stay on track.

ACTION STEPS

The more you know, the less you fear.

We all have some fears, doubts and worries when we are making a change. Fear of the unknown is one of the biggest hurdles in effecting enduring change. But these factors exist only until we choose to respond to them with the necessary actions.

The first step to making this change is to accept these emotions and take action any way. The more action you take, the less fear will exist.

The same is true of feelings of discomfort, anxiety and distress with regards to the healthy changes you make in your life. When you know what you are feeling, you can respond by finding the basis for that feeling. Eventually, we can remove the negative impact of that particular emotion by removing its cause. *Once we understand the source of these emotions, we can reorient our mindset to respond to them. And then they will no longer form these barriers in our path.*

Action Exercise

There are 3 key elements to change, each of which is essential for lasting change. Let's go through the process of understanding these steps and then apply them to the world around us.

The first element of all change is a*wareness*. If anything, I hope the first part of this book helps you to become more aware of what may be holding you back from the changes you desire. We need to be aware of *what we do* in order to change it. We can become aware by watching our actions and by becoming conscious and curious; by observing our thoughts, emotions, beliefs, habits and interactions with others, while paying attention to them. This will help you to respond appropriately to situations, circumstances and events in your life by tapping into the full range of your potential, rather than inappropriately reacting to events driven by thoughts, fears and insecurities of the past.

The second step is *understanding*. True understanding is the recognition that you can make all the changes necessary to obtain all the results you desire. I'll repeat: **You must understand that you possess the power to make the changes necessary for the life you want**. You are not helpless, hopeless, incapable or ignorant of what it takes to succeed. Your awareness and acceptance of this truth, once applied to any situation, will fully equip you to acquire the life you desire.

With this awareness, seek to discover and understand what your thoughts, emotions, habits and choices mean to you. *What do these factors mean to your success, your wants, your goals and your aspirations? What meanings are hidden and how do they hold you back from success?* Once you are able to see the aspects of your conditioned habits, you will be better equipped to change them or replace them with more healthy habits.

Finally, the third step is finding a *solution*. If we know what we do and why, and we understand that we have the power to change it, we are then able to find a way to replace unhealthy habits with healthy ones. Depending on the specific issue being addressed, different solutions may be necessary for different problems. Unhelpful eating habits, like eating too much, can be modified by reducing portion sizes. Eating unhealthy foods can be replaced with eating healthy choices. Physical activity and exercise habits can be modified as needed.

Some situations are best avoided or planned ahead; others may require you to seek the advice of others. The trick is to find a solution that leads you closer to your goal without creating a new problem in its wake.

Let's follow some of the main areas that we need to develop awareness about, understand the problem and find solutions. Do remember that this process can take some time and it is important to respond to each problem that you find. Consider this time as an investment in getting to know yourself and eliminating/changing the known and unknown from impacting your goals.

Resetting The Mindset

Awareness – Write down what you saw, heard and experienced around health, food, weight, dieting and exercise from your childhood. Watch yourself and observe your thoughts, beliefs, emotions and actions. Study yourself to be able to see your programming and conditioning for what it is. This will help you understand how your *mindset* was formed as you grew up, and how it holds you back.

> For example, when I was growing up, I was always asked to eat more helpings and finish everything that was on my plate. With time, this caused me to suffer from portion distortion, and automatically reach for more helpings of food that I liked. To eat even if I was full, until I had "finished all my food."
>
> I still tell my clients today to eat until you're satisfied, not until you are stuffed. Because I can remember back then, that I was only satisfied when I was stuffed – lesson learned.

Understanding – Knowing what led to the habits helps us in making sense of how these learned choices play a role in our present day lives. Write down how you believe these statements have affected your current lifestyle so far. Also write down how they affect your everyday choices about food, weight, dieting, and exercise. Can you see that this conditioning is not who you are of your own choice, but who you learned to be? Understand that was your old way but you can choose a new way ahead that is better suited to your health goals.

Continuing the example, when I realized that I was sabotaging my own health by the way I showed my appreciation for food, I understood that I had the capacity to choose my responses to these situations. I could find ways to show my appreciation that did not involve overeating.

Solutions – Knowing why you do what you do can be freeing in itself. The next step is to find an alternative course of action or response to people and situations that hamper your progress. Know that you can consciously choose to release any belief, emotion or habit that is not supportive to your goals, health and lifestyle. This is where you can start reconditioning your *mindset* to develop new beliefs, thoughts and actions. Think outside your comfort zone to find a suitable response. Ask yourself, *What actions can I start today that will move me towards my goals? What choices will keep me moving forward rather than backwards?*

Continuing my example further, I learned to balance my meals and to slow down my eating so my hunger could catch up to my fullness, since I was a very fast eater. I also taught myself to spread out my eating during the day, and take smaller portions each time, particularly when I knew that I wanted to try different dishes. This way, I am now able to please my taste buds and express my joy without having to overeat.

Understanding Emotions

The pivotal role of addressing our actions, is to understand the emotions that cause our actions, either overeating or eating inappropriately. The following three steps can be applied to reviewing our emotional responses as well:

Awareness – Keep a journal of everything that you eat on a daily basis but also add in what you were feeling when you made the choice to eat something. Be conscious of your emotions and what emotions are causing you to eat. Look for emotional triggers and become aware of which foods you consume when you are responding to that emotion.

For example, I have one client who would turn to chips in response to feelings of irritation about work. Another client craved sweets strongly during PMS. Knowing that these emotions of irritations and frustration triggered their food choices was the first step to changing that response.

Understanding – You can choose the meanings you ascribe to your emotions. If you are an emotional eater who is self-sabotaging your results, changing the meanings of these feelings can help you respond differently to the situation. Understand that you can choose your thoughts and thereby regulate the emotions you feel.

> For example, the clients mentioned above, tried to understand what caused their emotions/feelings in the first place. While the first realized that self-doubt and fear of failure were driving her, the second realized that her emotions were a result of trying to ignore her body's needs. This knowledge helped each find effective responses to their problems.

Solutions – Think of constructive actions and thoughts that can help you replace the meaning you give to your emotions. Make a list of these new actions and try each one until you find good/appropriate responses. Sometimes, a different response is needed for the same emotion in different circumstances; be flexible enough to find this response. Although this is a tedious process initially, it soon becomes just another habit over time if practiced.

> Continuing the example, the lady who was having a bad day at work chose to use affirmations that helped her feel more in control of her work. She also reached out to a

trusted colleague to discuss her work related doubts – a strategy that not only helped her feel better, but also better perform her job. On the other hand, the second lady learned to accept that she needed to treat herself but consciously chose healthy, comforting snacks and portions that she could turn to and reduce her desire for unhelpful foods.

Assessing Your Environment

Too often, the barriers for our chosen helpful behaviours are external. Unless we know how these factors play a role, we are likely to be met with disappointment in reaching our health goals. Take some time to identify what aspects of your environment are supporting you and which ones are holding you back.

Awareness – Take an inventory of what triggers exist in your most familiar environments – home, workplace, transit, etc. Identify if the cues you receive prime you to succeed or set you up for failure towards your goals. Explore your television habits and your socializing. *What healthy options can you incorporate into these environments? Alternately, can you reduce the impact of unhealthy options available to you?*

> The example I will use here may resound with many of you. Many clients of mine would take a lot of effort to eat healthy, but

> when they met up with their friends on the weekends, they would feel obligated to eat a lot of unhealthy foods. For the most part, they felt afraid of insulting their friends or making them feel uncomfortable.

Understanding – You have to understand that YOU must control your environment or your environment will control you. And you can control your environment. This is a lifestyle change, a lifestyle choice, not a diet, so things will happen that seem out of your control. You have to make space for unplanned foods and events and you have to plan the rest of your meals and activities according to what is best for your health. Fill the most common places you would eat with healthy options and remove all or at least most unhealthy options if you can.

> My clients from the above example realized that a lot of this unhelpful snacking happened because they did not discuss their health plans with their friends and family. Thus, they decided to inform them of their decision to lose weight and gain health and how they could help them in the process with these outings.

Solutions – Buying the right/healthy groceries and fresh foods is the best place to start, to bring in and surround your kitchen and home with healthy foods makes it easier to reach for them. Plan and prep ahead of time – this will save you time in the future and will give you some "go to" already made foods when you find yourself busy. Buy healthy snacks, but find and look for things that you enjoy eating. Find time and schedule exercise regularly so that your body receives the training that it needs. Tell people around you about your decisions and find solutions to common events that could impact your choices.

> Continuing the example, my clients made a conscious decision to choose healthy options even when eating with friends. If you look for healthy options, you will find them. If they had some foods off their plan, they made sure that they had a plan to get right back on track the next day. Also on most occasions, they started to eat healthy meals before going out to parties, etc., to reduce being tempted.

PART II

The 6 Fundamentals

Principles To Create A Successful Lifestyle Change

It's *Choice*, Not Chance, That Leads To A *Change*

#1. - The Principles Of Choice For A Lifestyle Change

In the first section of this book, we discussed how a lifetime of unhelpful habits, thoughts and actions, have held us back from success. We know how our *mindset* and our comfort zone influence our choices in food and exercise; in trying to safeguard us, they inadvertently hold us back.

We also reviewed how all these factors – our *mindset*, our comfort zone and the *wall* around this comfort zone – are learned behaviour. This means that we can *unlearn* them and learn new ones, which are more helpful and conducive to life's opportunities and constraints.

You are aware how your past conditioning influenced your past and present actions. What you may not realize is *past conditioning does not have to determine your future*. It is true: all your past choices – about food, exercise and your health – may have yielded less than adequate results. But you can change as soon as *you make the decision to change*.

Now is the time to make a choice: <u>Will you make the necessary change(s)</u>? Will you start this journey of unlearning old patterns and learning new ones? Will you decide to push through the discomfort, and pay the transition costs that are a part of changing your comfort zone?

If your answer is YES, you have made the first and most important step. You have chosen change over familiarity. This change will touch many aspects of your life.

On this journey, we will modify your lifestyle through thinking differently, mastering your emotions and creating new behaviours that will give you the results you desire. We will consciously take steps that bring you closer to healthier choices, which will lead you to develop a healthy lifestyle including healthy habits. This, in turn, will help you maintain your health long term.

Choices equal results. When I gained my weight, I did it by choice. I say *by choice* because the food I ate did not accidentally go into my mouth. I chose to eat it, despite my awareness of the impact it would have on my health. When I chose not to be mindful – when I chose not to live a healthy lifestyle or be physically active – it was the same as choosing to gain weight.

Similarly, your daily routine is the reason you weigh what you do. It is all the small things that add up to the results that you've been getting. But, just like myself, the moment you choose to eat healthy and exercise regularly, is the moment you choose to get closer to your healthy lifestyle goals.

The Power Of Choice For Life Change

We are the architects of our own bodies, built on the choices we make.

The physique we have is built on the choices we make. This means that we can build ourselves into the physical entity that we want to be. Everyone has their own goals – some may prefer to be lean, while others want to be muscular, etc.

Whatever your goals may be, being healthy should be at the top of your list. But, for either result, we have to first choose what we want our ultimate goal to be. Making a conscious choice is the first step, and we are doing that now.

Conscious choice, by itself, is a process. It starts with having an idea of what changes we want, followed by making a decision and committing to make the change. We have to choose what thoughts we want to hold onto and which ones to let go of.

We have to decide what to pay attention to, learn to modify the way we think and analyze the actions we take.

There are 3 types of choices you will have to make to create a life change:

#1 - The Choice Has To Be Yours

Choice is internal. Conscious change does not come from external prompts; it comes from our own awareness, thoughts and choices. The choice to change only works if YOU make the choice for yourself.

We have many people in our life who can inspire and motivate us to change – like doctors, partners, parents, friends, and co-workers. While all these people can become our support system and help keep us going, they cannot make the choice for us. They may want to help, but YOU are the one who is going to put in the work, deal with the discomfort and power through the emotional highs and lows (a natural part of change).

This is one of the biggest things I learned throughout my work: change is internal and it starts with you and your choices; no one can do it for you. For my clients, whenever the choice was made by others, my clients did not maintain *their* goals. Initially, they might have believed that they needed to change, but could not go the distance because the choice was not their own.

Similarly, I can show you the path, but YOU must be ready to walk down it. I can empower you, but YOU must find and slay your own demons. First, you have to understand that this will not be easy and you must be ready to take on the hard, consistent work involved.

What I *can* promise you is, if you take this journey, you will get the results you desire. If you understand your starting point and are crystal clear about your goals, then you will find fulfillment at the end of this process.

The real first step is to be 100% sure that you want to do this AND are ready to commit to the process. You must be 100% mentally, physically, and emotionally ready, to face all the fears, anxieties and roadblocks that are the by-products of the undoing of your old conditioning. At times, you will feel overwhelmed; if you stay the course, you will find the strength to excel over time. Note: long-term success and loftier goals require much work; this is a process.

Clearly Define What You Want

Internal choices are personal: start on the right path by clearly defining what changes you want and need to make. Would you tell a taxi driver, "Just take me anywhere" or would you say, "Take me to the mall?" Taking you "anywhere" will run up a bill you wouldn't believe. "The mall" could be any mall; the driver cannot assume you want to go to the nearest. See the amount of confusion and the costs involved without the right language?

Your lifestyle change(s) and goals are no different; it is important to be very specific about the changes that you want to make. These choices should be based on your ideal future self and should describe all the ways that this future self is different from who you are now. "I want to be skinny" is not a great way to describe your future self. "I want to be skinny" is a vague, non-specific definition.

On the other hand, "I want to weigh *x* pounds," "I want to run a marathon" or "I want to get off a certain medication" are good goals because they are measurable. Remember, all the choices that you make today will shape who you become. This means that you have to start making choices *today* that reflect your future self. If you keep making choices that reflect the person you want to be, you will become that person.

First, start by being crystal clear about what you want and where you are going. **Being vague will leave you with vague results.** If you do not know exactly where you are going, you will find it difficult to make the choices to get there and to stay there. Otherwise, you will end up giving up and never finishing what you start. The change you desire requires the strength to weather the storm and the uncertainty that lies ahead.

Take a long hard and honest look at where you are today. Write down the things that you want to change. Make a note of what specific changes you want for each aspect that needs to change. What are the differences between you and the person you aspire to be?

It's tempting to start talking about the steps needed to become your future self. We will come to that point soon enough. None of these exercises will help if you don't have an accurate idea of where you are today, and where you want to be, in six months, in one year, in two years, etc.

What do you want to change?	What does your change require?
1. Self love	Self love mindset
2. appearance	Control
3. Weight	maintaing my path
4. confidence	all of the above
5.	

You Today	vs.	The Best Version Of You
1. Overweight		– change my mindset
2. unhappy		
3. cheating myself		– work on self talk – positve
4. trying but not trying		attitude for change
5.		

Get Leverage

Another key to making a successful lifestyle change, is knowing what aspects of your changes will make you happy. Be clear on what you want to accomplish and why. Answer the question, *why will these changes make me happy?* Knowing the answer is one of the most important pieces of information you need to start the journey in order to leverage this opportunity.

Leverage puts you in the driver's seat: it allows you to *use something to maximum advantage*. For example, if I gave you $50,000 to invest, would you prefer a return of $150,000 or $300,000? Most, if not all, would immediately answer $300,000! Even if a financial advisor were to guarantee the return of either choice, the amount of work and risks required would be totally different. A triple return versus a six-fold return, will have entirely different strategies, deadlines, risks, commitments, options, etc. Your health and lifestyle changes are no different.

Look at your list on the previous page. Look at the desired changes you listed and what you said it would take for those changes. (*You may want to complete those exercises again.*) Now look at the present YOU vs. the desired or better version of yourself. I have already informed you that <u>the physique you want is built on the choices YOU make,</u> h*ow bad do you want it?*

If you want to sustain a lifestyle that takes you towards your goal, it is important that it makes you happy. Knowing what will make you happy in the process, will be the driving force on your journey. This is pivotal in the battle to create new habits and shift your *mindset*.

The next question to ask is, *Why do you want to change?* Find all the possible answers for why you want to achieve the goals you set:

Why do you want to do this? *health, self love*

Will it affect the way you feel about yourself? *proud*

Will you be healthier? *yes!*

Will you have new experiences that are currently not possible, due to your health and weight? *yes!*

Knowing your motivations, and understanding your intentions, will help you justify your efforts on days when you come up to *the wall*. We have discussed how moving out of your comfort zone will produce doubts, anxieties and fears. Answering these questions BEFORE starting the journey, is one effective way of ensuring that these doubts and anxieties will not weaken your resolve and make you give up.

Next, consider *what will happen if you don't change?* Doing nothing, staying where you are, may appear to be the easiest thing to do. But what will happen as time passes? How will you feel about your present self in five years or longer? How do you feel about yourself today, for the things you didn't do years ago, which is why you have the body you see in the mirror? Now don't think I'm trying to give you a guilt trip, that's not my intention. The past is what it is, the past. It's about planning for the future and understanding yourself and your motives. If you do nothing, will the situation worsen and lead to more weight gain? Could you suffer a weight-induced health problem like a heart attack, diabetes or arthritis? Will your excess weight affect your relationships (i.e., your body image, self-esteem or feelings of self-worth)? These are the answers that will steadily remind you that you can not give up. They are deterrents to reverting back or quitting.

Think of the future and the risks you face if you *do nothing*. Many people wait too late to make a decision about their health and only start being serious about it after they have a health crisis. Although many people are able to take these second chances as a wake up call, others might not live to. Preempting these problems, and using these risks to keep you moving forward, can save you and your loved ones a lot of trouble in the future.

Example: My father was a smoker for almost 50 years and was trying to quit for about 10 of them. One night, he suffered a heart attack. Fortunately, he was hospitalized in time and operated on, resulting in marginal damage. On that day, he made a decision. He chose to quit a 50 year habit and never looked back. Although I hope that everyone gets the opportunity to recover from such illnesses if they strike, I know that everyone does not get a second chance. Some wake up calls, you don't wake up from.

Make It Important

Your healthy lifestyle changes have to be important enough to YOU. If not, you won't do what's necessary to follow through when things get tough. One of the biggest mistakes people make in lifestyle changes, is focusing on the *transitional costs*. They don't focus on what is truly important to them, the reasons why they needed to make changes in the first place.

We can easily go back to our past behaviours and accept unpleasant, less desirable results because that option is easy. Many times people give up on diets because they are tired of coping with their emotions and the stress of doing things unwillingly. This is why we need to understand what adds to our happiness, as well as what subtracts from it, and make it a priority. We have to make our health a highly valued, priority goal and know why bettering it, will make you happy.

Now you have reasons to move forward on your journey and to not give up. Now you have reasons for change. Remember to find answers that are important to YOU. If the answers are things that others tell you, or things that you think you should value, but really don't, then you will find it hard to consistently follow through towards your goals. Remember, change comes from YOU.

#2 - Make Choices Outside Of Your Comfort Zone

How can you make choices that will lead you to your goals? *By consciously choosing to do things that are outside of your comfort zone.* One by one, you will learn new choices and habits that pave the path to your future, ideal self. Your body is built one choice at a time – each one just a little further from your present comfort zone and just a little closer to your future self.

Think of it as a maze puzzle: your present self is the starting point and your future self is the goal. You have to take small steps, one after the other, on the correct path that takes you to the goal. Similarly, you have to make small, incremental choices that will take you towards your future self. No Olympian or celebrated athlete, arrived at that status overnight. When you see their wins and celebrations, you also see the fruits of hours and years of hard work, consistent training and persistence.

Dr. Brian Wansink finds that the average person makes approximately 250 decisions about food every day. Although that seems like a lot, this means that we have just as many chances to move out of our comfort zone. We cannot take any of these choices lightly. Each choice, if correctly taken, will lead you a step closer to your desired goal. On the other hand, every time you give into your past *mindset*, you move your goal just a little further away.

We all want to be healthy, but making that choice, on a consistent basis, can be a challenge. The temptations are many and standing strong takes effort. One way to help you make better choices is to make a list of them, and use that list as a cheat sheet, for moments when you are tempted to fall into old habits.

What are these better choices? They actually fall into a range. There are many options that can be healthy, depending on where you start out and what your goal is. There is a lot of documentation – in books, on the internet and different programs – on healthy eating, how much to eat and on exercise. Choose alternatives that are best suited to your life and work constraints, your dietary needs and restrictions and your likes and dislikes. You may want to try a healthy diet program that you have done before or ask a friend or professional for guidance. Armed with this book's knowledge, you are now setting yourself up for success in any healthy endeavor.

Sticking to healthy choices can be tough; many of you know that from personal experience. The real problem is that when we make extreme changes, a lot of them are not *livable*!

The important questions when choosing a nutrition and or fitness plan are:

To the best of my knowledge, is this healthy?

Is this livable (not for a day, or week, but for the rest of my life)?

How often have you heard it said, "I cannot wait until this diet is over so I can go back to eating like I used to eat"?

This is why most diets do not produce long-term success; if you do not make permanent changes, the results will not be permanent.

You Are Still You

Permanent change scares us. Many of my clients resist change because they feel like they will lose a part of themselves. They worry that they will become a different person. It is necessary to keep in mind that, although these rules can be applied to making any behavioural changes, we are only talking about food and exercise.

Yes, you have to learn new ways of thinking about food and fitness, but your core personality will not change. If there are some things that you truly enjoy eating, there are always ways of incorporating them into your lifestyle and any healthy eating plan long term. A healthy lifestyle only changes the way you *indulge* in these things.

Consider that your present ideas of indulgence are governed by your current *mindset*. If you change your *mindset*, as we plan to do during the course of this book, your ideas of indulgence will change. You can still enjoy the same items, if you still like them, but in ways that do not harm you. Perhaps, if you leave your old conditioning behind, you will also find that you like some new foods more and some old favourites less. If and when this happens, it will not be a forced change; it will be organic and based on the extent to which you enjoy various foods. And, indeed, you will find that you will enjoy eating foods that give you energy and make you feel better.

Success is all about being honest and clear in your reasons, and making them important enough to you, to continue to strive forward in the direction of your goals along your journey. If you know why you are making a change, and you emotionalize it, you will succeed. Success is rarely easy, but – with concentration, dedication, awareness, and discipline – it is within everyone's grasp. For someone who is ready to put in the work, it's all a matter of time.

> *Integrate who you are with what you want.*

Setting Challenges

Every choice that falls outside your comfort zone, is a challenge that you have to overcome. When you set challenges for yourself, you should follow the elastic zone rule. Elastic Zone Rule: the challenge should be difficult enough to stretch you out of your comfort zone, but not so difficult that you stretch too far and just snap back into old habits. The idea is to choose goals that are difficult but manageable.

Achieving goals gives us a sense of accomplishment that fuels our efforts. Nevertheless, we need to consider the days when we are less motivated, and establish manageable goals that we can keep. If the better version of yourself requires major changes, it's important to focus on a series of process goals, versus solely the result goal.

> *When motivation is high, stretch further. When low, stretch less, but keep stretching.*

Making choices outside your comfort zone will make you feel uncomfortable. This discomfort is your transitional cost. Try not to focus on these transitional costs, but focus on the benefits your new lifestyle is giving you.

Most people focus on how uncomfortable they feel in their new actions and quit as a result. They forget about all the benefits that are coming with their new healthy life choices. This is the result of paying more attention to the negative vs. the positive; the temporary moment of pain or inconvenience vs. the future pleasure. Keep making new choices outside of your comfort zone and you will get new results.

#3 - Committed Choice To Change

> *One of the hardest things to do is to truly commit yourself to a routine – to new habits, to a lifestyle – that are all new to you. It is also one of the most rewarding.*

DOUBTFUL DIETING TO LASTING LIFESTYLE CHANGE

Most of us just like to "try things." We often want to "see" if a diet or exercise fad will work for us by embracing the short-term results. We don't like to invest too much time in it because we feel that it may not work as well as we hope for. But real and lasting results only come from consistent, long-term efforts.

Difference between someone who is committed to change and someone who is just interested

I distinguish these perspectives as a "Dieter" (*someone who is interested in losing weight*), versus a "Changer" (*someone who is committed to getting rid of the weight*). A **Dieter** is a person who is determined to take the shortest route possible to weight loss without planning for the long term. They go by what is effective and fast – from crash diets to cleanses – and **do what they have to when it's convenient.**

On the other hand, a **Changer** is a person who plans long term and commits to real change that is lasting and livable. **They do what is necessary to achieve this.**

How do I know when someone is just interested in losing weight vs. when they are committed? I look at their actions. Someone who is interested in losing weight, but are constantly overeating or eating unhealthy foods, will not put in the required effort such as physical activity. People that are interested, or pretending that they want to lose weight, just hope that it will happen but never really put forth much effort to change. They will not do what is *necessary* only what is *convenient*. When obstacles arise, they run back to their old, bad habits and poor decisions (comfort zone).

On the other hand, when you are committed, you take the necessary daily steps to progress and move forward regardless of convenience. You focus on lifetime changes and are willing to be patient enough to achieve them.

Three Stages To Change

There are three stages of change, each more effective than the previous one. These are three incremental stages that lead to success:

I want to change

I choose to change

I commit to change

Wanting change is the first and least involved step. This is where people want the change to come to them. This rarely happens so they are left with long-term dissatisfaction.

Choosing to change comes next, and is more effective, because it involves an active and conscious desire for change. These people are likely to put in more efforts, but are easily discouraged.

Committing to change. Real, long-term change comes only when one commits to change. It is not enough to want and choose change; you must *commit* to making the effort required for change. Those who commit to change know that they need to be patient, as well as consistent, in order to fulfill their goals. These people do not accept failure, but power through any temporary discomfort to achieve their goals.

Today, I want you to commit to change.

I want you to accept that your desire to change and your choice to take the effort towards that change, are the building blocks for starting this journey. I want you to commit to finding the path that serves you best, and following that path, until you break out of your old *mindset* and establish a new one. I can promise you that, if you make the commitment to change, everything will change for you. If you make healthy changes, your health and future will change.

The Secret To True Commitment

When you are truly committed to this process, I assure you that you won't even see those unhealthy foods that you think you need. Your focus will change from thinking about the things that you shouldn't eat to thinking about the things that you should eat and how to incorporate them into your lifestyle. You'll go from overwhelming temptation and cravings to a natural craving for healthy food choices.

True commitment has three key ingredients:

- Taking 100% responsibility

- Changing your rules

- Taking daily action

People who do these three things consistently are truly successful because they are committed to changing their lives and to the associated process.

1. Taking 100% Responsibility

The first key in becoming truly committed to the process is taking 100% responsibility. When you accept responsibility, you accept ALL the consequences of your actions and choices. Only you can make the required long-term changes in your life. Your future success will be built on your present actions and decisions. Your success will depend on you believing that you are in control of everything – your environment, your thinking, your emotions and your responses.

Of course, you cannot change the way people think, but you can change who you spend time with and who you listen to. You can completely control your thoughts and behaviours. Taking 100% responsibility is knowing that, no matter what happens to you, you control how you will respond. No matter the circumstances, situations or events that happen in your life, you are in the driver's seat.

DOUBTFUL DIETING TO LASTING LIFESTYLE CHANGE

If you are going to be successful, you have to take ownership. You are the one who creates your environment and creates what you think and feel. You create your results by your actions. Successful people believe this; unsuccessful people believe that everything just *happens to them*.

My successful clients face most of the same challenges that the unsuccessful clients do. The real difference is that the successful ones choose what they pay attention to and how they respond. The unsuccessful ones allow their environment, other people, and other factors to exert control of their personal choices and responses.

Remember: YOUR body is a product of YOUR decisions and not your conditions. The day you choose to take 100% responsibility, and refuse to let any situation affect your decisions in a destructive way, you will start rapidly moving towards the success you envision. Allow yourself to trust that you have the tools, resources and resourcefulness to create your own future. And don't allow anyone to tell you anything different!

I had a client, who was 77 years old and quite overweight when she came to me. She had already had two heart attacks and open heart surgery. She needed to lose weight, but her doctor told her that diets didn't work. Her doctor didn't think that she could lose the weight at her age.

This client chose not to give up, but she was unsure of what to do. She had tried a lot of diets in the past and knew that she had to do something different. When she first came to see me, I reassured her that she could lose the weight and change her life, regardless of what anyone said or her age.

I reassured her that she had complete control and power to change, and I drafted a plan to start her on her journey. Over the next year, she not only lost the excess weight, but became healthier than she had been in years. I will always believe that this client's journey to success started the day she chose not to be disheartened, to take 100% responsibility for her health and never give up.

> *You can't choose how people treat you or what they say about you. All you can choose is how you react to it.*

When you take 100% responsibility for your life and decisions, you feel powerful. When you feel powerful, you effect change. Ask yourself, *who is the real writer of my life's story?* It is you, but if you don't believe this, you may be falling into one of the following five traps, that keep people from taking full responsibility and staying committed to their goals.

Trap 1: The Excuse Maker

Some people tend to excuse their efforts and use difficult moments for reasons to give up. Many of us don't even realize that we are in the habit of doing so and that, by using excuses, we are sabotaging our goals. We love using excuses and often become very good at making them.

I was great at making excuses for my own weight gain and why I wasn't doing anything about it. But in order to lose weight, I had to lose all my excuses. Unfortunately, a lot of my clients found some of them and picked them up.

Many of our excuses sound legitimate until you stop to consider what you can do about the situation. The most common ones I've heard are: "I'm too busy," "I have no time," "My genetics are against me," and "I'm too old." I can assure you that none of these are valid.

I have had clients of all ages and conditions – people with multiple illnesses and people whose work consumed most of their waking lives. If the client prioritized their health, they succeeded. Those who used excuses did not.

There is never a time management problem, only a self-management problem. You can have results or you can have excuses, but you can't have both. If you are looking for one, you can always find an excuse. Or you can find a way. Remember, it is possible to plan healthy lifestyle changes, whatever they may be. It doesn't matter how crazy your life is. If you really want to do it, and you are committed, you will be able to. You have to be stronger than your excuses.

Around the start of my practice, I started making a list of the excuses my clients told me. I came up with a list of over 40 excuses. Over time, I realized that my clients who used excuses, failed; not because they didn't want results, but because they gave themselves an *out* from trying too hard. The biggest problem with the list, I remember, was that the client wasn't on it. The list was made up of situations or circumstances that were happening around them, but they didn't take any responsibility for their responses. Remember, *change comes from you.*

When you are reassured or comforted by your excuses, you will not feel the urgency to succeed. Each time a client comes to me with an excuse, I inform them that the excuse holds them back from success. I ask them to choose between success and their excuse. The ones that let go of their excuses succeed.

Trap 2: The Victim

The victim never believes that they do anything wrong; they blame their lack of success on everyone else. How can you spot a victim? Two ways: 1) they are always **blaming** something or someone for their health issues or 2) they are **complaining** about how things keep happening to them that won't allow them to be successful.

> Blame: Blame puts the responsibility of the situation squarely on something or someone else. But it also gives away your power to change, by implying that you are incapable of controlling the situation. Think about it:

DOUBTFUL DIETING TO LASTING LIFESTYLE CHANGE

> Why would you change if it's not your fault but someone else? You wouldn't.
>
> Complain: Complaining is a way to deflect responsibility that assumes that external circumstances are more powerful than we are. Complaining can make us feel good for the moment, but it makes no positive change in our lives. It eliminates the courage to push for what we want despite the situation. Complaining means that you have a picture in your mind better than you are willing to work for.

For example, when I was overweight, I blamed my parents, friends, and school, as well as my genetics. It took me a long time to understand that I was able to control my own choices and that blaming others was not helping me change.

I remember two clients I had during the early years of my practice. One was a mother of two young children; she always complained that her hectic schedule kept her from eating right. At the same time, I had another client who was doing very well, despite of having seven young children. When I asked her about how she managed to stick to her nutritional plan, even though she spent her entire day taking care of her children, she said:

> *I do not find it hard at all to eat right and to stay healthy, because I never want to look at my*

> *children and think that they are the reason why I am not healthy. I always want to look at my children as the reason to be healthy, to be fit so I can be a role model of health and achievement for them.*

The first client was blaming her situation; the second used a far more difficult situation as her inspiration.

Many of us are in the habit of blaming the people around us for the situations we find ourselves in; we complain about what is happening in our lives. In doing so, we forget that regardless of what happens to us, we can choose how we respond to the situation.

You can't change the people around you, but you can change yourself and your decisions. Taking responsibility for your responses and choices will open up a lot of doors to change. Know when you start hearing yourself complain or blame your current situation, circumstances and events for your health, they will start to close.

Trap 3: The Procrastinator

These are the people who plan for the future, but do nothing today. They always plan to start their exercise or diet the next day, next week or after some event ends. They always have a reason to do something later and love the word "someday." They say things like, "Someday I will lose weight," "Someday

I will eat healthier," and "Someday I will go to the gym." *Someday* is code for *never*. By the time the start date arrives, they find another reason to push it further.

The best weight loss procrastination device is Monday. How many times did you fall off your diet and say, "I'll just start back on my diet on Monday," even if it was only Wednesday?

What we never realize is that life never gets less busy. There is always something waiting to take up your time, and unless you keep your goals as a priority, you will never find it at the top of the list. The procrastinator has good intentions, but has trouble starting things.

If you procrastinate, take a moment to realize that you will never find the 'perfect time.' But if you push yourself, and start on your journey, you will find a way to incorporate your healthy choices into your life and start to get the results you want.

One of the biggest procrastinators I met was a young woman in her 20's. She had an active social life, but worked a demanding job. She had been putting off prioritizing her health and losing her excess weight for years. When she came to me, she was full of ideas about what she would do next week, next time she bought food, next time she went out, etc. She knew what she had to do but just kept putting it off.

I gave her goals that she had to complete each week. When she started to do the things she needed to do, she began to see the results she wanted. After finding out how easy it was to get started, she wished she did it sooner. Slowly, she abandoned the habit of procrastinating and experienced remarkable success. She was shocked by how much she achieved in a few months after coming to me. After all, she had been dealing with her weight for years while she procrastinated. Even if you just start with little goals, start there and start now if you are a procrastinator.

Trap 4: The Rationalizer

Similar to the excuse maker, the rationalizer tries to explain away their failures and lack of effort. They tell themselves *rational-lies:*

I fell off my plan because I had to eat out.

I had to eat poorly because I had people over.

I couldn't exercise because my work increased.

Rationalizers don't feel too bad about failure because they have a logical explanation for it. But rationalizing their failures and their lack of effort simply blocks them from taking more effort, from finding the correct regimen and trying again at something they gave up on.

Rationalizers believe their own stories. Do you find yourself giving up on your rules only to be able to explain the situation? Then you may be rationalizing. The only way to break out of this habit is to make success non-negotiable. Tell yourself, "This is not optional," each time you see a rationalization coming up. Do not allow yourself to explain the situation, either to yourself or to others.

A client I had used to rationalize his lack of exercise by citing his crazy work hours. He had to learn to stop using rationalizations before he started seeing the opportunities to exercise, stay active, and to eat healthy, that accommodated his work hours. And the moment he found these opportunities, instead of telling his *"rational-lies,"* he started seeing results.

Trap 5: The Justifier

The justifier is a person who has learned to minimize the extent of a problem. They live by the statement, "It's not so bad; it could be worse." The moment we start thinking of how much worse something could be, we start to feel comfortable with the way things are. We become complacent for things not being as bad as how we imagined.

This is a protective habit that tries to spare our feelings. But thinking of how things could be worse, distracts us from planning for how they could be better. It's great to be grateful, and gratitude is one of the most powerful emotions. But when you focus on how much worse it can be most of the time, instead of how you want it to be, there is a problem.

Taking Responsibility

The only way to change your habits and your life, is to take responsibility for the existing circumstances. Maybe external factors have played a role, but at the end of the day, you are responsible for your weight and healthy state. Others in your life may have been responsible for conditioning you from a young age, but YOU are responsible for change.

Reality check: it is your responsibility to keep fit. It is your responsibility if you feel that you have no time to find the time. Similarly, it is your responsibility if you're in the best shape of your life! You are responsible for that. Just like it's your responsibility to plan ahead and to prepare food and to fit exercise into your schedule. Just like it's your responsibility if you are reading this book and taking action, realizing that your life doesn't ever have to be the same again.

We have to take responsibility to change our thoughts, change our environment – add new friends, read different books, watch different shows, and to do whatever it takes – to put us on the path to better health and keep us there. The idea is to reprogram ourselves to think at a higher level to produce the results we want.

When you take responsibility, you realize that you have the ability to change your response. You start to analyze all the reasons why your efforts did not work in the past. You ask questions like: *What was I thinking? What was I doing? What was I eating? What was my emotional state? What were my actions that produced those results?* When you start to ask yourself these questions, you begin to find answers that will help you in responding to situations, circumstances and events that happen in your journey.

Using a meal log or journal can really help you with this process. This can be the start of your learning experience about you and your eating habits. Learning from past mistakes is the best way to ensure you don't repeat them.

A meal log or journal helps you figure out what's going on. This is a book in which you write down all the things that you eat, drink or exercise – meals, portion sizes, snacks, additions made to the meal, any fluids, as well as any exercise. It helps keep you accountable to yourself. Simultaneously, it also creates an awareness of what situations and triggers produce unhelpful eating for you.

Once you identify your triggers and eating patterns, you are ready to make changes to them. Don't think of the meal log as a representation of your guilt; think of it as a tool that will help you find the things that you can and want to change. I recommend keeping a meal log no matter what plan you are on, as it allows you to identify all your eating habits and trends. This will allow you to see what you are doing and review your "responses" to certain events, situations and circumstances, when you are not getting the results you want.

2. Change Your Rules

The second key in becoming truly committed, is that you need to change something and that is changing some of your rules. We all live by a number of unspoken rules. These rules define our habits – from the time we wake up and what we wear, to what foods we choose and what activities we partake in. Most of us are usually unaware of the little rules we have for ourselves, until we pay attention to the *musts* and *shoulds* that we follow.

> For example, your body is a representation of your rules. *Are you fit?* If so, I'm sure you have a "rule" to exercise several times a week. *Are you muscular?* If so, I'm sure you have a "rule" to do weight bearing workouts several times a week, etc.

Become aware of these "rules" and then make corrective changes for achievement. Make new, non-negotiable rules for yourself – ones that will take you closer to your goal. Find ways to stick to them long-term. Making rules for how you live is an essential part of long-term change. You are not truly committed to your health goals until you change something, and when you make yourself a rule it is much more than a choice or a should, it is a must for you.

These are rules about how you live. These rules will form your baseline behaviour and will prove to be your saviors once you get to the maintenance. These rules, which will be habits by then, will ensure that you stay on the path of healthy living for the rest of your life.

Choosing Rules

Clients often ask me what kind of rules they should make. I tell them to make rules that will help them be healthy, regardless of their life circumstances. The following are just a few examples of healthy, positive "rules" that you can incorporate into your life:

A morning walk

Doing some sort of exercise 30 minutes a day

Prepping meals and snacks ahead of time

Finding healthy eating options when you eat out

Not eating unhealthy snacks right before bedtime

Reading books that encourage you to be active and healthy

Eating a specific portion size for meals

Eating breakfast

Sleeping from 7-8 hours a night

Making sure that you are getting enough water a day

It takes some time to get used to these new rules, but this is also the time when you are learning to develop a new *mindset* that will compliment these. Know that there will be days when you break one of your new rules. Use that as a learning experience and move ahead, ensuring that the situation that caused you to break your rules is understood and responded to. This is a lifestyle change not a diet. Things will happen. Move on and beyond.

Sometimes the simplest of rules can turn your life around. One of my clients was a lawyer who spent half the month traveling because of his work. In a few months, he found that he was gaining a lot of weight from the food choices he was making when he ate out while traveling. When he realized that this had also happened to another senior colleague who was on the road a lot, he made one simple rule for himself.

He decided that, no matter where he traveled for business, he would choose healthy, balanced meals in the restaurants he visited. He soon realized that the restaurants did have healthy options when *he looked for them*. This simple rule helped him rapidly lose the weight he had gained.

Consider the people in your life. Some will be fit and healthy, others not so much. If you just observe the choices made by each person, you will find that the fit person typically seems to have habits and rules that encourage their fitness. The unhealthy ones will have habits and rules that contribute to them being unhealthy.

On the face of it, the healthy, fit individuals may seem blessed with a naturally lean body or great metabolism, but this is not the case. It's the person's rules that they live by that makes them fit and healthy. The person makes healthier food choices and/or exercises daily, in order to maintain their health and fitness.

They become fit because the rules that they live by are tailored around them being fit. Similarly, you can contribute to your developing health by designing some livable rules that will encourage healthy choices and healthy living. Make these rules non-negotiable for yourself, regardless of the situation.

Responding To Others

When you first change your rules, people around you will have to adjust to these new rules. They are used to the old you and it may be uncomfortable for them initially. Some people will adjust to these; others may try to change you back to the old ones. It is your job to stand firm at this point and continue making the conscious new choices that you are making.

Friends and family can feel uncomfortable if they feel judged by your new rules. It may help to sit loved ones down and explain to them what your rules are and how you plan to apply them to your life. This may help them understand your motives and support you. If someone does not want to support you, choose to spend time with them in situations where your new rules don't come up.

Remember that these are just *your rules*; not the rules of your partner, your family, nor friends. Other people must be free to live by their personal values and rules. Explain the idea to them, and if someone wishes to join you on this part of the journey, make them feel welcomed.

But if someone prefers to do something different, you need to let them do so while you keep to the habits you are trying to form. Remember, it is OK if one friend orders a burger and fries and the other orders a salad at the same table. Live and let live. It doesn't matter if they need to lose weight or have poor health, you cannot choose for them. When your rules start showing results, some people will see the value in them and join you. Whether they do or don't, continue on *your journey* to health.

3. Make The Effort And Take That Action

The last key in being truly committed to your own health and goals is to *take action on it*. Initially, it will be difficult because your body will not be used to the new choices and rules. It will demand the foods that it is used to, and the activity level that it is comfortable with.

But it is now your job to act on the choices and the rules you developed, and translate them into daily and weekly behaviours. Initially, you will find yourself full of excuses and reasons to skip the new and healthy choices, but you have to make yourself follow through as much as possible. With some discipline, you will find yourself getting used to these new choices and behaviours as they start to become habits.

Action is the link between your commitment and your results.

When you start taking action to change your life, remember the *5P's: patience, persistence, perseverance, positivity* and *permanent*. First, you need to have *patience* with yourself. It will take time to get used to following these new rules and taking action on these new choices.

You have to be *persistent* with your new behaviours for them to start showing any results. Note: these results may initially be slow to come by. You will have to *persevere* through the bad days – the emotional highs and lows and through all the doubts – before you can be assured that you are on the right track. But taking this effort will definitely yield you long-term results.

To keep you from giving up, you have to think *positive* thoughts. Be kind to yourself and trust the process. Finally, remember at all times that you are aiming for *permanent* change. Incorporate changes that you can live with.

Remember: A new body just doesn't show up; it comes from within, built on the daily choices you make. You are the architect of your own body.

Final Words

I want you to wake up every morning, excited about your health and lifestyle. Start making healthier choices as soon as you get up; feed off that momentum for the rest of your day. Do this every day, as much as you can. Use your past results to learn about which of your choices caused them. Your future results will be built on the actions that you choose to take today. Take each day, one decision at a time.

Each decision comes down to the moment when you are making them. The choice whether to have dessert tonight, may seem insignificant, but it is not. Is one dessert going to ruin your ability to achieve your weight loss goal? Absolutely not. However, if you keep eating in a way that does not support your journey/goals, this one decision becomes more and more significant. Decisions made in the moment are very significant because this moment, is all that we have. The choices we make in the moment, must be based on who we want to become or we never will succeed.

The decisions you make when you are alone, when no one is watching, allow you to find out who you really are. Not only that, but you see a preview of who you will become. Ask yourself, are you making choices based on who you want to become or who you were? Once you know the difference, you will know how to shift your *mindset* to reach your desired goals.

Use every moment to your advantage; something may seem insignificant at the time, but every decision leads to long-term results. When you make the right decisions over and over and over again towards your goal, they will have a compound effect and start to build momentum. This is key to not only seeing results, but feeling the results as well.

Some days it may be difficult to make so many healthy choices, but if you persevere and motivate yourself, you will find the strength to get past the temptation. Choice is your power to use; use it to better your health and happiness. Your success starts with your decision to change, make choices out of your comfort zone and commitment to this change by taking 100% responsibility, changing your rules and taking action today!

So what is your change tomorrow? If you don't make changes, then everything stays the same. But the day you commit to make a change, is the day your entire life starts to change.

Action Steps:

Get leverage on yourself: Know that it has to be your choice. Make a list of why you want to change and what will happen if you don't. Make a list of what will happen if you do make these healthy lifestyle changes (each list should have at least 10 items). Hold onto this list for motivation.

Define what you want: You have to be clear about exactly what you want to change and what you are determined to do. Use specific, measurable language like, "I will lose 10 lbs." rather than "I want to lose weight." Next, make a list of the things about your eating habits and exercise that you will change to get you there. These lists are now your specific goals.

Make that commitment: You have to take 100% responsibility. For the next 30 days, there has to be absolutely no more excuses, blaming, complaining, procrastinating, rationalizing or justifying your mistakes. Accept each moment of mishap as it is and make a note of it. Use your meal log and use this information to fine-tune your choices. This will have a huge impact on your life.

Take action: Pick no more than three things that you can start doing now from step two. It has to be outside of your comfort zone, which will move you closer to the results you want. Start taking action on one or up to three goals today and do them for 30 days. When you feel comfortable with doing these consistently, pick another one to three goals and start them for another 30 days, and so on.

Focus In The Direction Of Change

#2. Principles Of Focus For A Lifestyle Change

Focus, *the driven attention that we pay to the things we are doing*, is the key to success. A person who is focused on his/her goals is the one who is going to succeed. I have found that, the extent to which people are focused on their goals and reaching them, determines their degree of success.

Most of us focus on dieting and not for life change.

Those who are crystal clear on what they need to do and are focused on how to achieve it, take the additional effort that most goals demand. These are the people who break out of their old *mindset* and form new habits that are effective.

You have to get clear on your core values and what you want to accomplish. This is really the only way you can rise above the negative chatter and the self-doubts that start when you challenge yourself. When you are not as focused, anything is a welcomed distraction from the effort that will take you to your goal. This is because distractions are easy, but your new lifestyle requires effort. Focus helps you see nothing but the result of that effort.

Are You Focused On The Wrong Goals?

Goals VS. Results

Most of us are focused on the wrong goals. Most people that want to lose weight spend most of their time focused on that end result. It is great to have an ultimate weight loss goal, but it should not be your main focus.

Think about your ultimate goal, write it down and put it away somewhere; don't worry about it anymore. This is where most people get it wrong. The biggest reason we lose focus is because the eventual goals we set for ourselves are daunting and often do not seem achievable. We are overwhelmed by how far we have to go, and then we get lost in the distractions that make us feel better for the moment. What we need to do is not think about the final goal, but to think of the daily process goals that will take us there.

It's great to have a final goal to work towards, but the direction it gives us is the extent of its value for us. It should be used as a guidepost to look at occasionally, but not as a daily measure. The people that change their lives, recognize that the goals that really matter are the ones that are part of their daily routine. They know that they have to focus on the process and make process goals that will yield the results they want, instead of just focusing on the end results they want.

> *Your final goal is the promise you make to yourself, your daily goals are your promise plan.*

Your daily focus should include the amount of exercise you have taken, the foods that you have chosen and the amount that you have eaten on any given day, etc. You have to focus on the fact that you want to become a healthier, fitter person and your ultimate goal weight is just a benchmark for becoming that person. Focusing on the process helps you do what is really important: taking the small, everyday steps that help form the habits that yield results.

> *If you focus on results, you will never change. Focus on the change and you will get the results.*

When you focus on the process goals, the emphasis is on learning and growing as a person. This means that you develop skills that will help you throughout your life and in various situations. But, if we make the mistake of focusing on just a target weight, we may lose a lot of this learning along the way. Focusing on reaching a particular weight will not necessarily lead you to become a healthier person.

Focusing on daily process goals also means that you are focusing on small, manageable steps that will likely lead to success. On the other hand, focusing on the final goal can mean that you are likely to become overwhelmed and give up simply because the goal may be so far away.

What I find in the weight-loss industry is that there is too much emphasis on results versus analyzing the outcome goal and organizing it into a lifestyle, process-oriented action steps. As a result, you never really learn or grow along the way. This attitude is what sets us up for future failure. How many infomercials, new and old, have you seen on weight loss pills and potions, which promise to help you "lose the pounds effortlessly and quickly"? Yet, you continually see new ones and the obesity rate is on the rise. Why?

Because none of these "quick fixes" emphasize learning or long-term, transformational behaviour. If you don't change your *mindset* and identify those factors that caused your weight gain/struggle, you will not have long-term success. This is not only true for "quick fixes" but sound programs as well.

Remember: while learning and growing equals results, the reverse is not true. If you just focus on losing weight, there is no guarantee that it won't come back. But if you focus on learning about yourself, your habits, your lifestyle, and how to change your life to lose the weight, your life will change so you won't revert back to the person that allowed the weight to pile up. It is ironic, but the only way to reach and maintain your goal weight, is to not over think it during the process.

Focus On Developing A Growth Mindset

As previously discussed, the biggest change that needs to be made is our *mindset*. If you have a *fixed mindset*, you have to focus on changing it to a *growth mindset*. People with a *fixed mindset* believe that they are the person they are and that their essence and habits cannot change.

They see failure as permanent and are more likely to give up trying, after a couple of failed attempts. On the other hand, a *growth mindset* is one where a person believes that they can keep learning and growing their entire life. This mindset allows them to see their failures as lessons and to keep trying new things.

I have found that people who come in with a *growth mindset*, or develop one along the way, are truly the successful ones. This is because the *growth mindset* allows them to be flexible and incorporate all lessons learned into their everyday choices.

Dr. Carol Dweck, author of the book *"Mindset,"* discusses the difference between the two. She says that the people with a *growth mindset* succeed because they see challenges as exciting, not daunting. They believe that they can learn and enhance their abilities, so everything is just a matter of time.

On the other hand, someone with a *fixed mindset* assumes that their basic qualities, intelligence, talents and abilities, are just fixed traits. That they just have a certain amount and that's it. These individuals are disheartened by a challenge and see that challenge as beyond their reach.

> *A growth mindset means the capacity for you to see your abilities, not as fixed, but as infinitely improvable.*

It seems obvious that we should have a *growth mindset* if we want to succeed. But more often than not, we fall into the trap of using a *fixed mindset*. The biggest problem this creates is that we stop believing that we have the ability to change ourselves and our circumstances.

For example, if you have a fixed belief that you are just an overweight person and that's the way it is, that belief acts as an excuse to avoid practicing good eating habits to lose weight. The *fixed mindset* prevents you from failing at smaller, individual attempts, but in the long run, it hinders your ability to learn, grow and develop new skills.

On the other hand, someone with a *growth mindset* would be willing to try and learn new exercises, new foods or ways to prepare it, even if they failed at creating a healthy lifestyle in the past. They don't give up until they learn what works for them.

There are clues that you are thinking from a *fixed mindset*. The most prominent clue is if you catch yourself saying or thinking things like:

I can't lose weight.
I can't work out regularly.
I can't change the way I eat.
I can't eat healthy food.
I was always big and I will always be this way.

When you find this happening, take a moment and reposition yourself to think from a *growth mindset*. Remind yourself that there are a lot of options, and if one plan does not work out, there are other options. As a health professional, I can assure you that there is a plan that will work for you. Remind yourself that habits can be learned and unlearned; you just have to find the right process that works for you.

Losing Focus

When the going gets tough, it's easy to lose focus of what is really useful. I frequently have clients who tell me that they are unable to stop thinking about past failures, what they are not supposed to eat, or about being overweight. I always tell them that the things that you focus on create the prominent themes of your life.

If you focus on your limitations, you will feel limited most of the time. Your journey will be difficult and will not make the required lifestyle changes. If you focus on why you can't or why you shouldn't do this, you will stop dead in your tracks.

Shifting habits consciously and creating reminders of success and positive habits, is necessary to maintain your drive and to keep moving towards your goals. You should focus on the present and the everyday choices that you have to make versus the past. You have to focus on what exercises work for you and what foods are good for you. You have to pay attention to the direction you are taking and the future person that you are becoming.

The more you focus on these things, the easier the journey will feel. It will also help you find the courage to learn new things and expand your options – something that focusing on your shortcomings will never allow.

What Are You Focused On

What you focus on most of the time determines whether you will succeed or not. I see this all the time with my clients. With the best of intentions, people still make mistakes in choosing what they should focus on. Our environment is full of distractions and experiences that do not support our goals for healthy living. But most of us tend to focus on these aspects of our environment, especially because it is right there in front of us. This is why we get tempted by advertisements and shows that feature food; why we feel inclined to try the latest fad that promises weight loss; and why we are frustrated when an exercise regimen that worked for so-and-so celebrity does not work for us.

These distractions are everywhere – on television and radio, on flyers and in the mail, in our newspapers and magazines. The brightest signs are displayed on fast food places strategically located on the busiest street corners, tempting us to take the easy way out of eating a healthy meal. Our friends describe fancy, rich foods in great detail, but rarely talk about healthy eating. It's no wonder then, that we lose focus so easily.

When you find this happening to you, make a choice to not be distracted. Choose health over distraction in your environment. Focus on making one lifestyle change after another that is livable and healthy. Focus on adding healthy foods to your diet and incorporating exercise into your lifestyle. To become the person you want to be, you have to focus on the choices of that person. You have to focus on how this person behaves and follow up on those everyday actions that will allow you to become this future you. <u>Every single day</u>, you have to be focused on the specific actions you need to take to become who you want to become. You will know you are doing the right thing when your focus starts feeling automatic and takes less effort than before.

We become what we think about, so let's think about the healthy, fit and happy version of ourselves so we can become that person. Developing a new *mindset* is all about focus and how to shift that focus. We have to focus on what we want and not on what we don't want. Caution: This is easier said than done, as we tend to automatically focus on the problems, obstacles and past failures.

I had a client who was stuck in her thoughts about her past failures and was demotivated about exercising. I asked her to create positive images and reminders to scatter throughout her living space.

The more she made herself think about the positive aspects of the future she was building, and reminded herself to do little exercises around the house, the less time she spent dwelling on the past. This meant that she spent less time worrying about possible repeat failure, and more time focused on the person she wanted to become and how to get there. Changing her focus allowed her to get past the initial habit forming period and eventually exercising regularly.

If you continually focus on what you want, you will move towards it. Most people focus on what they don't want, or what they are afraid of, which makes things too hard for most of them to move forward. Focus on what you want and you will find the energy needed to make it a reality.

Three Things You Have To Focus On To Create A Lifestyle Change

These are the three things that successful clients/people who make a lifestyle change tend to focus on the most:

The process

Solutions

The positive alternative to negative, unsupportive thoughts

If you can learn to focus on these three things most of the time, you will find that your journey is easier and more effective, in comparison, and has fewer hurdles.

1. Focus On The Process

One of the biggest reasons for failure are misguided ideas about what you should be doing. People make ambitious plans, but forget to consider their circumstances, the sustainability of the plan, and their limitations. As a result, they focus on drastic changes when they should focus on the small, consistent changes that yield big and lasting results.

You typically see this fallacy in the thinking of a dieter – a person who is just focused on losing weight and not on becoming healthy. *The dieter's mentality* assumes that reaching a certain weight will make him or her happy. On the other hand, a person focused on healthy, incremental lifestyle changes, thinks about how they can slowly mold themselves into a healthier person.

The lifestyle approach assumes that being overweight is usually the result of other problems, not the cause. Addressing these problems directly is the best way to solve both the problems themselves and the weight issues they cause.

What a dieter focuses on most of the time versus someone seeking a true lifestyle change, is vastly different…

A dieter focuses on just the results; lifestyle changers focus on the process.

You can lose weight by enforcing a restrictive diet and following it for one month or more. However, when you go back to your old diet and habits, you will soon pile the weight back on. You must be *in it to win it*; not for instantaneous results but FOR LIFE! By focusing daily on how to create a healthy lifestyle and how to incorporate this lifestyle into your own life, will give you results.

A dieter focuses on the foods they are not supposed to eat. A lifestyle changer focuses on what they are supposed to eat.

If you are constantly looking and talking about *forbidden* foods that you are *supposed* to stay away from, you will soon abort the mission and go back to the various habits and patterns that led you to the very place you are trying to escape/improve. A better approach is to eat according to your goals, which is more of a balance between best practices and results driven eating. To focus on the foods that are on your healthy eating plan and finding different ways to make them enjoyable.

A dieter focuses on the fastest way to lose weight. A lifestyle changer focuses on getting rid of weight by incorporating sustainable changes in their lives.

People who focus on making a lifestyle change know that, when they lose some weight, they need to make steps for permanent change. They know that they are moving towards having a healthier immune system, digestion system, feeling better and having more energy. They know that when they change their daily routine, everything else changes as a consequence. So they look for ways to make sustainable changes that fit into their day.

They focus on incorporating lifestyle changes that work for them while thinking long-term. They are concerned about the results but they don't focus entirely on just results. They work with an assurance that the results they desire are natural by-products of the healthy changes they make. The *mindset* of a lifestyle changer is focused on identifying the lifelong changes needed for permanent results. If you focus on change, not *quick schemes and gimmick products*, you will achieve the desired goal. If you focus just on results, which are often supported by *quick schemes and gimmick products*, you rarely receive the desired results or lose them soon after when you lose your momentum and drive.

The reason why diets generally fail long-term, is because the focus was solely on results (as fast and as easy as possible). Generally, diets do not encourage dieters to think about how, or if, the recommended changes fit permanently into the dieter's lifestyle. This is why, when your diet ends, you experience weight regain and you're back to square one.

Long-term change is hard; it challenges you to the core. It takes discipline. You have to be relentless in your quest for change and weight loss, but you must be balanced and flexible. I know, it sounds like an oxymoron and is an interesting paradox. Be clear about what you want and go for it, but if something isn't working (not producing the results you wanted), be able to switch things up and keep going.

Search for the process that works best for you. Never be afraid to seek professional help; often skilled, health professionals can quicken the process for you. Look for programs that are customized to each individual and his or her needs. They should provide a clear course of action that fits with your goals and lifestyle to best achieve the results you desire. Once they eliminate the guess work of what will and will not work for you, they can pinpoint what your next course of action should be – short term, in the interim and to the finish line (and beyond). The investment that you will make in hiring a professional can give ends to years of potential frustration, confusion, and failure.

Regardless of whether you seek professional help or do it alone, you have to ask the questions: Is this recommended practice/diet/program, healthy (to the best of my knowledge)? And, is this livable for me?

2. Focus On Solutions

There will always be challenges and obstacles on your weight loss journey. You can choose to focus on these problems or on the solutions. A person on a diet may worry about the problems; a person focused on making a sustainable change, will search for effective solutions. He or she knows that focusing on the problems won't make much of a difference, without possible solutions. Looking for a *way out* is a waste of time.

> *A dieter focuses on the obstacles;*
> *a lifestyle changer focuses on solutions.*

When you focus on your problems, your goals start to disappear. If you focus on your goals, your problems start to disappear.

Someone making a lifestyle change knows that obstacles will show up. They expect the obstacles AND they *plan* for them.

> *A dieter thinks one or the other;*
> *a lifestyle changer thinks*
> *they can do both.*

A dieter thinks they have to choose between the diet and life events. A lifestyle changer knows that they can find ways to balance both.

> *A dieter focuses on what they did*
> *wrong; a lifestyle changer focuses on*
> *how to move on.*

A lifestyle changer focuses on their health habits and learning to overcome obstacles. They don't get hung up on what they did wrong on the diet or what "treats" they shouldn't have had at the party. They know that their healthy habits will keep them stay on track, and what they do most of the time versus just some of the time, is what matters most.

> *A dieter gives up after a mistake;*
> *a lifestyle changer accepts the lesson*
> *and moves on.*

Small mistakes do not mean failure to the lifestyle changer; they are simply symptoms that need to be addressed. Those who understand this will use small, progressive goals to keep them on track. These small, progress goals are exactly what make lasting changes.

> For example, you notice that you've been eating a lot of fast food recently and have not gone to the gym in a while. You know you need to make better choices, but you have not addressed the issues that caused your recent changes. As a matter of fact, you've rationalized your behaviour because you say to yourself, "We all need a break, from time to time."
>
> Upon further analysis, you just received a promotion at your job. Although the promotion was a long time coming, the weighted blessing has produced feelings of doubt and added pressure. Your free time is almost nonexistent, in part, because you spend your every waking hour obsessing over what you can do better to enhance your skill sets and professional persona.
>
> Now that you know what the problems are, your short-term solutions can be: 1) make sure you have on hand, (at home and in the office), healthy, convenient food choices that

are quick and easy for you to grab on the go. 2) drink eight or more glasses of water throughout the day. Purchase a 1 or 2-liter water bottle and make sure that it stays by your side, refilling and drinking it throughout the day; and 3) walk for at least 20 minutes every day during your lunch break. These are small changes that fit into your high pressured lifestyle, with minimum disruption, that will help you lead to your desired health changes.

Whatever we focus on, we tend to get more of. If you continually focus on all the problems and obstacles you are facing, or will face, more and more will keep popping up. If you focus on the solution and how you can better your situation, you will find various options that will work.

If you find that nothing is working for you currently, give yourself permission to walk away and try again after you have addressed the other problems. In the meantime, you will have laid the foundation and developed habits that make it possible to tackle more complex issues.

Many people believe that they can't go out and enjoy themselves while on a diet. Lifestyle changers disagree and believe that having fun at social events is a natural part of life. They have the confidence that they can balance their new healthy choices with any event.

For example, let's consider going to the movies. The dieter will worry that the popcorn will affect his or her diet. The lifestyle changer, on the other hand, may choose not to eat the popcorn but will enjoy the movie. He or she may choose to have another, healthier snack or smaller portion of popcorn, as an alternative.

The latter allows these individuals to enjoy their lives, as they did before, and find ways to incorporate healthy lifestyle changes along with the activities they enjoy. As a result, they don't feel deprived nor resentful, and can sustain these changes because their overall emotional experience is a positive one.

A person that makes a lifestyle change is someone who knows that there will be mistakes and treats along the way. A person who makes a lifestyle change knows that they can have whatever they want to eat, but also knows that treats are treats. While treats alone are okay, they do not allow these "treats" to become habits, which creates other problems.

3. Focus On The Positive/Supportive Alternative To Destructive Thoughts

In saying this, know that you will have negative thoughts; we all do. But people who truly make a lifestyle change know that focusing on these destructive thoughts serve them little to no purpose. Lifestyle changers switch that focus to the positive alternative, constructive thoughts that lead to new actions. This is where personal power comes from. Let me state that again. When you focus on the positive/supportive alternative to a negative/destructive thought and take action on it, this is where personal power comes from.

> *Dieters focus on how they can't and why they won't. Lifestyle changers focus on how they can and why they will.*

Most of all, we have to change our internal, negative self-talk. Most of us are hoping positive, but thinking negative. Most of this is fed by our negative self-image and our environment, which has conditioned us to think in such a way. Some examples are:

> *This isn't going to work; I can't do this.*
> *I'm not worth it or I don't deserve it.*

Perhaps you embrace these thoughts because you have tried so many things before and failed. Perhaps someone told you that you couldn't do it and you believed them. You don't have to look too far for negativity when you are trying to make a life change.

You have to be careful how you talk to yourself because you are listening. I sometimes ask my seminar audiences: *If your best friend would talk to you as you talk to yourself, would they be your best friend anymore?* The answer is almost always *no*! That just proves the high amount of negativity that we place upon ourselves.

ANTs

Automatic Negative Thoughts, or ANTs, have been discussed a lot in self-help literature. ANTs are negative thoughts that we unconsciously practiced to the extent that they become second nature. They raise their ugly heads every time we try a new thing and they make us doubt our ability to ever change.

These are self-harming thoughts that hold us back, because they convince us that we are incapable of improvement and change on any level. ANTs can pass under the radar because they reside deep in our subconscious. An indication you have them is when suddenly you doubt your efforts, your choices and your ability to do something.

The first step to breaking out of their control is to recognize the negative loop you are stuck in, become aware. Next, consciously challenge these thoughts and break them apart logically. Does your ANT tell you that you can never change? Confront it with the question of whether you have tried this method before. Does it demoralize you by saying that you can't exercise? Respond by making a list of the things that you like about your new exercise routine and all the victories, great and small, that you have experienced already.

Initially, you will have to consciously take action against your ANTs each and every time. Soon you will find that your positive responses become more automatic; the negative thoughts become weaker. With time, you will replace the negative spiral with a positive, motivating one. Most of your negative thoughts will die from malnutrition, because you will no longer feed them time and effort. Not that you won't have the negative thought(s), but they will slowly stop winning each day.

Remember, the more positive your internal chanter, the easier it is for you to stick to your goals. So, regardless of how scary and painful it is initially, take the effort to affirm your abilities, your energy and your strength. As you begin to believe in yourself, you will find that you have more motivation and focus on the *right things*. You will be able to attend to your daily goals with greater confidence and increased determination that will drive you to complete the more difficult goals.

You can benefit from listening to motivational, inspirational messages daily. Sometimes we all need daily affirmations to override negative self-talk. As you slowly internalize these messages, you will find yourself relying less and less on the external source, but it's still a great idea to continually feed your mind with these messages.

You can find daily positive affirmations online, books, CD's or you can ask a trusted friend or colleague to verbalize the positive that they see in you. If you have hired a health professional for guidance, discuss your feelings with him or her. Surround yourself with positive energy and messages that instill confidence. Soon you will find yourself thinking in the same way. Avoid the people, or situations, that give you negative messages. Soon you will find that your negative self-talk becomes quieter and quieter.

To Help Stay Positive, Focus On Your Future Self

Successful people focus on their future self – and take joy in the person they are striving to become. These individuals pay attention to the habits and preferences of their future self. As a result, they incorporate these habits and choices more easily in their lives.

These people are driven by the knowledge that, the more they act like their future self, the sooner they will become that future self. On the other hand, people who typically lose focus tend to place more attention to the things in their past. They fixate on what they can't do anymore, on what foods and portions they can't eat and on what habits they can't practice.

The past is just that: you can't change it, go back or change any past events. The future is just that: infinite possibilities and room for anything you imagine and work hard to create. Fixating on your past, those things you can't do anything about, will keep you feeling tired, drained, dissatisfied and overwhelmed. This is why some people give up when faced with certain difficult situations – they just can't handle or make the space for any more disappointment and unhappiness.

People who focus on their future are looking at positive things – things that will help them, things that they can do and control. This focus allows them to remain positive, even in the face of difficulties and setbacks. On the other hand, the ones who are looking at the things that they can't do, tend to feel negative emotions more. They focus on the negative past experiences – things that they can't change, and this will hurt their future goals in life. Be the *lifestyle changer* who looks to your future self for inspiration; not a *dieter* who looks behind in distress.

How Do I Get Started?

Are you having an 'Aha!' moment and realizing that a lot of your past failures had to do with your focus? Do you now see how easy it is for you to think non-supportive thoughts? Now that you know what has to change, the next step is to learn how to focus on the right things.

The first thing you need to do is identify the situations in which you find yourself thinking negative thoughts. Observe your thoughts and the connected downward spiral; see what triggers these negative thoughts.

Once you know what specific negative thoughts you have, you can *consciously* replace them. Each time you find yourself thinking, *I can't do this*, tell yourself, *This may be hard, but I will find a way to do this*. When you find yourself saying, *I will never change*, replace that with, *I am changing slowly but permanently*. Replace each negative thought you have with a supportive one.

Hour Of Power

Include your positive reinforcements in what I call your *HOUR OF POWER*. I ask all my clients to practice an hour of power each day. It may start out as just 20 minutes every other day, but I want them to practice this eventually every day. This hour includes spending 30 minutes exposing yourself to motivational, inspirational, informational or educational material, to aid you in learning ways to sustain your efforts to become healthy. If you continually feed your mind with the good, only the good can come out.

For the remaining 30 minutes, do some sort of exercise/physical activity. I call this the hour of power: 30 minutes of innercise and 30 minutes of exercise. This is a total game changer if you practice this consistently. This Hour of Power has totally changed my *mindset* and my life, but more importunately my clients' *mindset*, when they incorporate this into their daily routine. As a result, they change the way they look, feel, think and talk about themselves.

You can start by incorporating the Hour of Power a couple of times a week, to your everyday routine. The more you learn to invest in yourself – mind and body – the faster you will find yourself moving through your process goals and towards the results you desire.

Remember that all the negative self-talk is the result of how we are programmed. Initiating change means you have crashed into the *wall* surrounding your comfort zone. When you start to leave your comfort zone, your past *mindset* will try to reel you back in. Realize that although negative thoughts are part of your conditioning, you are not bound by them if *you choose* not to be. Once you protect yourself with positive messages and break through this *wall* of self-doubt, you will achieve the *mindset* change that will lead to eventual success.

Recap - 3 Key Things To Focus On When Making A Life Change:

Process. You can have the best ideas/vision in the world; without a plan of action, you will never achieve it. You must look for a plan that works for you and your lifestyle. Focus on the healthy foods you are eating and find ways to make these foods enjoyable for you to eat on a daily basis. Focus on making sustainable healthy changes that fit into your daily routine. In addition to the plan that you chose to follow, you must realize that the journey is a process and you must be prepared to handle it as such. Without an honest assessment and realistic expectation, you are doomed for failure before you can get started.

Solutions. A lot of us focus on all the existing and potential problems that attending our goals have to offer, but what solutions do you have prepared to counteract them? Focusing on your problems without coming up with possible solutions puts you in a position of hopelessness and vulnerability. Focus on solutions that will not only help you today, but in the future when/if these challenges resurface.

Positive alternatives. Your focus/perspective is what will drive you and give you a second wind in the rough times. The process/journey to weight loss, especially long-term, is not easy. When you add past failures, fears, doubts, and preconditioned negative thoughts, your attempts at healthy life changes becomes an uphill battle. Flip the script with daily positive innercise and exercise, including the *Hour of Power*, which will make success inevitable versus defeat. Making choices from the lens of your "future self" will be a transformative.

How To Get Better Focused

The biggest mistake we make in getting focused is over analyzing the situation. Although you are fighting thoughts with thoughts and emotions with emotions, the real success is in keeping it simple. Don't try to fight too many demons at once; this will only fatigue your brain and cause you to lose focus.

Keeping it simple also applies to your actions. Doing too much too soon will overwhelm your body and mind. If you can make ONE effective change at a time, and stick to it, soon you will be well on your way to success. You would be surprised how the simplicity of a small change at a time, will build incredible momentum. Start simple and start small. Each small choice will add up to big changes in the long run.

Remember to be consistent with each of these changes. Progress, no matter how small or slow, is the key indicator that we are on the right track. When we have progress, it is easier to stay focused as we rest assured in our choices. When we have none, we start to question everything and lose focus.

A lack of progress also means that mistakes have been made in some of your choices. Always remain flexible in your approach and switch things up just a little. Keep adding small, regular changes and track your progress, great and small, to remain focused on the right things you find working.

Questions

The way we talk to ourselves has a lot to do with where we direct our focus. This is because the things we say, and the responses to those questions and statements, are what stay in our conscious and unconscious minds.

Questions direct our focus

We often question ourselves to see if we are going down the right path. We ask questions like:

DOUBTFUL DIETING TO LASTING LIFESTYLE CHANGE

Do I want to eat that?

What should I wear?

What should I get for a gift?

We also ask ourselves a lot of questions about our choices and actions, with respect to our health and related actions.

The kind of questions we ask define the way we think. Our brains are like a computer; if you ask it a question, it will give you an answer. If you ask a bad question, you will get a bad answer. For example:

Why am I overweight?

Why do I keep gaining weight?

Why am I not eating healthy?

Why does this always happen to me?

Can I really do this?

These kinds of questions are terrible; the associated answers make you focus on your weaknesses, past failures and anxieties. On the other hand, if you ask yourself questions like:

How can I lose weight?

What is going to make me happy?

What can I do today to move me closer to my goals?

What can I do to take better care of myself?

How can I make this happen, right now?

What do I have to do, or become good at, to achieve my goal?

You will end up focusing on the things that put you in a position of power; things that you can control. The above are great questions because they serve the purpose of directing your focus in the right direction.

Ask yourself questions that propel you into action. When you find yourself asking a self-defeating question, or one that makes you focus on the past or on your weaknesses, immediately change your focus. Asking questions like, *How can I turn this around?*, or, *What can I do about this?*, will instantly refocus you to dwell on future actions versus pitfalls. The answers will give you the positive momentum needed to overcome current circumstances.

Use the ability of a question to create doubt to your advantage. Ask questions about the things you want to weaken. For example: maybe you realize you have a limiting belief that you find is holding you back. Ask, why do I believe that? Start questioning that belief. When you search for answers, a lot of time you will find it doesn't have any "legs" to stand on. Ask questions that challenge your old *mindset* and that weaken your old conditioning. Use questions to weaken the *wall* and to help you lose some of your old habits.

Language

Another way to get – and stay – focused is by paying attention to what you are saying to yourself and others. We already talked about positive/supportive thoughts verses negative/non-supportive, but also be careful about the words you use in your self-talk. For some, the word *diet* creates images of starving and short-term results. Substitute words like *lifestyle* to shift the focus onto actions that are enduring.

Be careful how you label things; your labels will determine how much you covet them. When you separate delicious food from nutritious, you are telling yourself that you can have either but not both. Instead, focus on using the words together – tasty, delicious and nutritious food.

When you find such a tasty, nutritious dish, don't say: *I can't believe something this tasty is healthy for me*. Say instead: *I'm so glad that something this tasty is healthy for me*. The first statement assumes that it's rare that healthy food is tasty; the second assumes that you can find more such options. When you say the second statement, you create a focus on food that checks both boxes and encourages you to look for additional dishes that are similar. Likewise, instead of thinking about the *costs* of becoming healthy, talk about the *benefits of having made the effort*.

> *You have to be ambitious about being nutritious.*

Watch your language. People that are just interested in losing weight, use words like *should* and *but*. I call them the *Should But* people; the ones that say things like:

I should go for walk, but . . .
I should eat healthier, but . . .
I should lose some weight, but . . .
I should eat breakfast, but . . .
I should drink more water, but . . .
I should go to the gym, but . . .

The list can go on and on. The word **should** acknowledges what has to be done to achieve your goals; yet the word **should** is the pause button to your goals. The word **but** is the stop button in goal achievement; it is the goal killer. The word **but** justifies why you shouldn't go after your goals; it gives excuses of why your goal is not worth it to you.

Equally as dangerous is the word *someday*. **Someday** is code for never; its cousin is the word **can't** which also means won't. If you hear yourself saying the words *should, but, someday*, or *can't*, immediately change your language. Once you change your language, your *mindset* starts to change. These words are all putting your goal achievement on hold.

Use the word *goals* to represent your direction, your daily processes that are going to build the ultimate results that you want to get. Use the word **promise** instead of *result goals*, *end* *goal*, or your *ultimate goal* that you are trying to achieve. The word promise is a lot more powerful then the word *goal*. Think about it. We always make goals for ourselves but we rarely make a promise to ourselves. Think of your daily goals as your **promise plan**.

If you want to make true lifestyle changes, you have to turn the word *should* into *right now* and the word *but* into *action*. The word *someday* needs to be replaced with *today*, and the word *can't* into *I can and I will*. Make that *promise* to yourself, and make a *promise* plan to get you there. Take action today. You already know what you should be doing; commit to doing it, right now.

Final words

Our focus determines what leads us. The key is to focus on what is truly important and what is going to make you happy and healthy. Say no to everything else. Choose to focus on what matters – your health and quality of life matters. Use your attention to think about actions and possibilities instead of conflicts and weaknesses.

Do not get upset about the body you have; get excited about the body that you will have. Don't focus on where you are today, but where you are going and your future self. Focus on the feeling of accomplishment and achieving your desired outcome.

Anything that you focus on for a consistent basis, you will achieve. Use this awareness, to focus on health, nutrition and exercise. Don't focus on the *transitional cost,* but enjoying the benefits.

Counter the negative self-talk with supportive, constructive statements that will bolster your spirits and serve as inspiration. Activate your focus by using the right kind of language and asking yourself the right questions. I promise you that, if you do this, you will start to see the endless possibilities instead of the hurdles; the potential instead of the risks.

Action Steps:

Focus on the process: Each time you catch yourself focusing on your ultimate result goal, substitute the thought with thinking about one of your process goals that will get you there. Instead of thinking, *I have 30lbs to lose*, think *I will walk for 20 minutes today* and then do it.

Hour of Power: Start incorporating the *hour of power* into your life. Start with 20 minutes, three days a week, and work your way up to one hour a day. For example, split 20 minutes between 10 minutes of innercise – reading, listening or watching something motivational, inspirational, informational or educational – and at least 10 minutes of physical activity.

Stop non-supportive self-talk: Pay attention to your self-talk during the next 48 hours. Write down all the negative things that you find yourself saying. Identify the top 10 and come up with supportive replacements. Use this list to replace negative thoughts whenever they arise. Then, for the next 7 days, go without saying or focusing on anything you know is negative. This will initiate the desired change in your life.

Ask the right questions: Make a list of questions that will keep you focused on process steps. Include questions like, *What can I do right now to help me get rid of this weight? What will make me happy? What will make me healthy?* Write down as many answers to these questions as you can, making a list of at least 20. Then start to act on at least one to three answers today.

Find solutions: Take a sheet of paper and write down all your long-term goals. Make two columns under this: in the first column, make a list of all the reasons that you haven't achieved these goals in the past and reasons why you think you may not achieve these goals now. Then, in the second column, write down all the action steps that you will take to counter each of the points in column one. If you find you don't have the counterpoint, seek outside opinions or conduct further research.

> When you find the answers, write them down. Start canceling the first column by listing its counterpoint. When all the items from column one have been countered, rip up column one and throw it away. Keep column two and focus on that. This exercise should help affirm to yourself that all doubts and problems do have solutions for you to follow.

The Motivated Diet, Eat With Purpose

#3. The Principles Of Motivation For A Lifestyle Change

One of the most difficult-to-find ingredients in the recipe for success is *sustained motivation*. A lot of us start on the journey to weight loss, but few finish it. It is estimated that over 95 percent of all weight lost from any given diet, doesn't last for more than two years. And a big part of this reason is that people do not have the motivation to push themselves forward.

People give up on their goals, or fail to complete their weight loss programs and stop maintaining their new healthy lifestyle, simply because they are not motivated enough to take the effort. It is difficult to tap into enough motivation to change our lives completely. When we lack the desire to keep going, to keep looking until we find the right solution(s), we give up and stay stuck in our old *mindset* and comfort zones.

Anytime we do something that requires a tremendous amount of effort, our success is deeply linked to our levels of motivation and our ability to sustain that motivation. It takes a lot of energy to deal with the people, situations, circumstances, temptations and events that try to hold us back. Motivation can provide the energy to keep pushing forward.

If you have enough motivation, it will drive you to overcome your environmental challenges, events, circumstances and inner conflicts that we all face in this journey. Consistent, strong motivation will turn your *maybe* to a *must;* an *I should* to a *right now*. Motivation is what will eventually help you create the habits you need to develop and find pleasure in healthy choices, and eventually, your healthy body.

Knowledge only has potential power; it is worthless unless you use it. A plan can put you on the right track, but you will need sustained motivation to keep you moving along this path. A coach or a trainer can guide you, push you, inspire you and demand success from you. But you, and only you, can motivate yourself to do what is necessary daily (and consistently) towards your goals.

So how do you develop the type of motivation that drives you every day? It's easy to do when we are young and not completely conditioned by outside forces. Have you ever seen an unmotivated baby? Of course not; they are motivated to do anything. As babies, we quickly learn from the world around us and apply that knowledge to create our initial *mindset* and comfort zone. Let us see how we can tap into the unbridled motivation and energy of a child and harness it with the discipline learned over the years.

The strongest motivation comes from inside us. External factors may help inspire us, but true motivation has to come from the inside. Many of my clients come to me for motivation, expecting me to provide them with a reason to take the necessary effort. But I can only inspire those who are already filled with the desire to change, and then give them an action plan to follow coupled with tools to sustain that motivation.

The same can be said about family and friends. They can push you, encourage you and support your efforts, but only you can make the difference. Your desire to complete the transition from your present self to your future self, is key to making the change. A sustained change in behaviour is achieved only when the motivation to do so is elicited internally by you.

I see my life as an opportunity to teach my clients, which now includes you, how to motivate themselves, so they don't rely solely on external forces. This will not happen overnight, but with a little time, you can find the right internal motivators to deal with roadblocks and obstacles. Remember though, I can help ignite this fire, but only you can keep it burning by fuelling it on a daily basis.

Motivation is like deodorant: for it to work, you have to apply it daily.

Cultivating Motivation

Motivation doesn't come overnight; you have to plant the seed and nurture it, until it grows into a strong force capable of propelling you into the future. The process starts with the idea. The idea that you are going to change your life and then you have to add emotion to take action. You have to define the change in clear, precise terms, so that you know exactly what you are aiming for. Once you know what you want, in clear and precise terms, and you are focused on what it is that you want, you need to find the motivation to fuel you to launch you forward.

What is *motivation*? Motivation is literally *the desire to do something*. It is possible to make motivation a self-feeding system that uses the thoughts and results of your recurring efforts to renew itself. What is important is finding something that you desire so deeply that you are ready to take all the efforts necessary to reach that goal.

You need to find a goal that inspires you, gives you hope for a different future and is real enough, that it fills you with determination. Together, these positive emotions can help you respond to all the negative emotions that will try to hold you back. Each time you hit a *wall*, you have to counter that negative emotion with a positive one. You have to fight emotion with emotion: fear vs. hope or anxiousness vs. excitement, doubt vs. determination and worry vs. inspiration. The more often you pitch a positive/supportive emotion against a negative emotion and win, the closer you will find yourself to your goal with a new *mindset* and a new future.

Personal, emotional reasons are essential at the start of the journey and throughout, because on the dark days, they will serve as a light to guide you towards a healthy result. A personal, emotional reason has to be something so strong that it overrides all your doubts simply because you want it so much. This is vital because your journey will have some transitional costs like we discussed in the first section. At the point when you are experiencing discomfort and pain, only your motivation for your future will keep you from giving up.

Our comfort zones are to blame. Designed to keep us safe, our comfort zone also serves the biological purpose of defining the activities that require the least effort. Our brains where designed to survive not thrive. This makes taking different daily actions/strides so difficult. Our habits are formed to reduce our efforts and now we are expecting ourselves to suddenly take a tremendous amount of effort on a daily basis.

Think of the "*wall*" as your home's exterior and the comfort zone as the inside. You are safe from all types of weather as long as you are on the inside, but this also confines you to this comfort zone. One day, you need emergency help but you are unable to move. You place a 911 call for someone to hurry up and come help you.

When the ambulance and rescue workers arrive, they don't politely tap on your door or softly push against it. This is an EMERGENCY situation! They team together, using a battering ram or tools necessary to break the door down and get to you. A gentle tap on the door or just one worker attempting to break it down would result in an extensive amount of time to get to you. Your home's door metaphorically represents all your anxieties and fears. To rid you of them so you can get the emergency help you need, they must be attacked with a battering ram. The "*wall*" must be weakened so you can break free immediately and get help!

Your motivation has to have the strength of a battering ram; this is an all out war! A small hammer simply won't do. Let us now take a look at your hammer-sized motivation and turn it into a battering ram.

There Are 3 Pillars To Cultivating Your Motivation

1. Your Vision/Body Image

The first pillar in building motivation is the vision or the body image you hold for yourself. Our brain works in images, so let's see how to harness that to our advantage.

The first thing I want for you to imagine is your desired body image at your goal weight. What do you look like? Find a picture from your past, if you have one, or of someone you admire; that will help remind you of your ideal body image.

Too often, we are stuck in the present because we allow our mirrors, clothes, and other things to define how we see ourselves. We adapt to seeing ourselves as the overweight, unhealthy mirror image; we easily lose vision of what our future self will look like. Reminding yourself of this future image, will fuel your efforts. Knowing the difference between the person in the mirror and the person in your mind, will guide the direction of your efforts.

Now I want you to imagine the rest of your life in this future – or at least the habits that surround your health choices. What does it look like when you are making healthy choices? What does it feel like to be the future you? It can take some time to build this vision; you will need to think of action after action, then you will need to re-envision them as they will be performed by the future you. How does this new vision make you feel about the future?

Over time, many of us condition ourselves to doubt our ability to change. We think that we cannot become fit, eat well and lead otherwise healthy lifestyles. We don't remember that we have done it before, even if it was short term; we do know what success looks like. If you are working so hard that you cannot envision or taste the future that you are working towards, it will be extremely difficult to keep your goals.

Give yourself an image to focus on; envision how you look and how your actions look. This image encapsulates all the things that you want and it shows you what you can become. Images are events in the brain and the brain cannot distinguish between what is imagined and what is real. A well imagined vision of your future automatically becomes an anchor for your efforts, by providing you with an event to look forward to. And this is the first part of building your motivation.

I can remember when I participated in my first bodybuilding competition. I used to have a picture of a bodybuilder that I cut out of a magazine. I thought I could look like him if I trained hard and dieted. I carried that picture around with me in my wallet all through the process of preparing for the competition. I did this as a reminder of what I wanted to become. I would see it every time I opened my wallet. That was a big part of the process. It was a reminder that, if I keep working hard, I can achieve that physique too. It was my first bodybuilding competition and I placed 1st in my class. I'm telling you this to reinforce the power of having a clear picture of where you want to go, and make sure you remind yourself daily.

The clearer your vision of the future, the more likely it is to come true.

There are many ways to create the vision of your future. Use older pictures of yourself when you were at your goal weight. Perhaps you have pictures of you wearing an outfit that symbolizes your goal state/weight. There are even software tools that can manipulate an image to the desired weight and fashion that you request.

You can use pictures of friends or family who have achieved successful weight loss as motivation. You can use pictures of celebrities and celebrity trainers, who advocate for healthy living and healthy habits you respect and admire. The only rule here is to know what you want and use an image to represent that desire.

When we have healthy lifestyle goals, often we tend to focus on images of the things we are trying to avoid – like unhealthy eating – or things we don't want to give up to fulfill our goal. We picture all the sweets and desserts that we *shouldn't* eat. But the moment we start to focus on these items, we are more tempted by them and our vulnerability increases.

How many times have you looked at that state you're currently in, and focused on what you would have to give up in order to achieve what you desired? Sometimes the thought alone is overwhelming and causes you to give up before you can even start. When we think of healthy eating, instead of picturing the benefits, many of us think of all the things we are going to try to avoid like sweets, chips, pop and all the "forbidden foods." This doesn't give us a very compelling picture of the future, nor does it motivate us to change. What we need to focus on is a picture of our healthiest self, followed by what actions are necessary to get there.

Instead, focus on the *do's* – what foods you are going to eat for your new healthy lifestyle, what exercises you want to do, etc. The clearer your vision is about the things you want to do and accomplish, the easier it will be to stick to these choices. The less you think about the things that you choose not to do, the less likely they will distract you and weaken your resolve.

If you have been overweight your whole life, or you don't remember ever being fit or at your goal weight, operate out of imagination and not out of memory. Envision yourself at your goal weight. Envision yourself becoming who you want to become and what that would look like. *How do you feel when you picture yourself there?* Thinking about the way we will feel about something can be a powerful motivator, since we want that experience to be our reality.

When clients come into the clinic for the first time, I look at their goal and ask them to think about the last time they were at goal weight. I ask them to remember how they felt. I ask them to build the image that they recall or create one from their imagination. This is a hugely important step to take, since it gives a specific vision to chase.

Often we are unaware of the body image we hold of ourselves and the visions we create. Some of us naturally create visions of our obstacles and eventual failures. Others automatically create visions of success and how they will look when success is achieved. When we create visions of failure, we feel unable to create visions of success. If this is happening to you, push

DOUBTFUL DIETING TO LASTING LIFESTYLE CHANGE

through that image and try to see yourself at your goal weight.

Envision how you will feel when you reach that goal. Is there anything more important than how you feel? No. Use all five senses to cultivate how you will feel. Remember, when we focus on one of these conflicting visions, the other fades away. You need to concentrate hard on the idea of the *successful you* to banish the idea of *failure*. Use your vision of your future emotions – your feelings of happiness, achievement and satisfaction, to guide you past any ideas of failure, fears and anxieties.

While you are creating this body image and these visions, remember to visualize real, livable changes. Create a body image for how you want to look three months down the line, then how you want to look six months down the line and so forth. Know that each vision achieved is a step towards an eventual goal. Think of how these future versions of you behave and start those behaviours today.

Ask yourself, what are the top 3 things that are really going to change in my life? Sit down and write them out. What's really going to change once you become healthier and fit? Paint a detailed picture in your mind of these answers. How are you going to look in photographs? How are you going to look playing with your children and/or grandchildren? What kind of clothes will look good on you? Which of your present clothes will you look much better in? And finally, while you are doing all these things, how do you feel?

Remember, your *mindset* is like a guidance system. For it to guide you in the right direction, it needs to know where to go. And this is where the vision of your future self fits in – the goal that you want to reach, and where your mind must take you in order to achieve it. Your vision is step 1 in developing motivation; it is your map of where you want to go.

When I decided to lose weight, I quit seeing myself as a friendly, 181 pounder and started to see myself as a friendly 150 pounder. I looked at pictures in magazines of people in shape. I gave myself a goal that I would look similar to those pictures. That is what helped push me along.

I had a client who had gained weight slowly and was initially unable to envision herself without her excess weight. I made her look for old photographs that represented the fittest period of her life, and asked her to make a collage of those pictures. She focused on things like how her body looked, what her measurements were, how she felt, etc. This drew up a detailed image that she used as her template for success.

I also asked her to keep a couple of favourite dresses from that time, to use as motivation. Every few months, she would try those dresses on, but not to focus on how tight they were. Her only focus was on whether the clothes fit better, even if it was only slightly. In five months, she was wearing the dresses she wore prior to gaining weight.

When you set a new body image for yourself, you basically acknowledge that you don't want to be where you presently are. You are aware of the difference between where you want to be and where you are – and the dissatisfaction over the difference after comparing the two adds to your motivation. Once you add this dissatisfaction to excitement for the future, this will inspire you to change. This is what happened in my previous example, when my client used past clothing to fuel her motivation.

What future results you visualize will be reproduced by your body. What you picture in your mind is so critical to your success; you cannot out preform your own body image. If all you can see is yourself being overweight and out of shape, you will not have the inspiration to push forward. Your performance will improve only when the image you have of yourself improves.

Your vision is your map, it gives you inspiration to move forward.

2. Your Expectancy/Beliefs

The second pillar to building and sustaining motivation is your expectation of your future – your belief in yourself. The expectations and beliefs that we hold are what drives us. Our beliefs determine what we consider acceptable choices and actions; our expectations of ourselves determine how much we will push ourselves and in what direction.

As your vision is your map, your beliefs are your guide.

For example, someone who believes that he or she will be able to complete a puzzle, will take extra efforts to find the right solutions. Someone who believes that he or she is bad at puzzles, or believes that solving puzzles is a silly activity, will not take the additional effort to complete it. They simply have no desire to do so.

Similarly, our expectations of how we will behave in different situations, as well as our beliefs about what behaviours and choices are available to us, will guide our health behaviours. You have to believe that you can overcome the hurdles and reach your goal. Your expectation has to be that you will fulfill ALL your short and long-term goals. If you believe that you can, the chances are far higher that you will. If you believe that you cannot, you won't put in the effort necessary to follow through. Whatever you believe will become your reality.

The mind produces your expectancy, which then manifests in your reality – your life and your lifestyle.

Our minds are primed by the beliefs and expectations we have. They naturally tune out all information that is not consistent with our belief system. If we want something bad enough, every experience becomes coloured as an opportunity to make it a reality. Thus, if you don't believe that you can make a lifestyle change, you won't. But if you believe in the change, it will happen for you.

Once you believe, you have hope; once you have hope, you have options. John Maxwell said it best when he said, "*When you have hope for the future, there is power in the present.*" Hope leads to finding actions; it becomes a part of your guidance system. But if you have no hope, then its game over; you will not achieve what you want. Why start something that you know you are not going to achieve? If you believe you will fail, then you won't try or will quit soon after. Making a half hearted start will not lead to a lifestyle change.

So many of my clients have lost all hope, and belief in themselves, by the time they come to see me. They have tried so many times before to lose the weight and to change their lifestyle, and have been left with disappointment every other time. My first job is to build that hope back up – not for a day or a week, but as a strong, driving force that will keep them focused on their goals.

You may have a compelling vision for your life, but if you do not actually believe that you can obtain that vision, you will give up the moment the first obstacle shows up. If you don't *believe* that your vision is going to come true, it won't. This is why it's important to have a realistic and attainable goal.

Breaking Through Old Expectations

A belief is our evaluation of a particular thing, which is made up of memories of our life experiences (or those of the people closest to us). The more we experience or have heard about this, the stronger our beliefs are. Our habits are guided by our beliefs; we determine right from wrong, and good from bad, based on our beliefs.

If you believe that ice cream will make you feel good, then you will reach for ice cream every time you feel bad instead of going for a walk. This is why we need to change our beliefs before we can expect to change our behaviours and choices. There is plenty of research to show that people who achieve their fitness goals are the ones who intensely believe that they can right from the start.

One of the biggest challenges to building helpful expectations and beliefs is that many of us are governed by the limiting notions we hold of ourselves. These limiting beliefs are based on our experiences and thus, are notoriously difficult to change. What has compounded your limiting beliefs? Take a moment to think about it. Have you tried many times before to lose weight and just couldn't do it, or maintain it? Now you have a belief that you will never be able to lose your excess weight? Has someone close to you told you that you couldn't lose weight, or change, and you believed them?

When you start thinking and talking about the things that limit you, soon you will recognize what has happened. You have to stop yourself and replace limiting thoughts with supportive ones. Remember, the only limits you have are the ones in your mind. To change this, you have to disempower the belief that feeds your doubt and hinders you. You do this by questioning it; start questioning beliefs that do not serve you.

Why do you believe _____? Are the supporting facts relevant now that you have started on this path? Remember, your past is behind you; you are trying a completely different approach to becoming healthy. By doing this, you start stripping the power away from your limiting beliefs.

Some of our limiting beliefs seem illogical or baseless, once we examine them. Most of the time, these are inherited from our parents, friends, associates or significant others. Recognize this and then strip their power by focusing on how baseless the idea or notion is.

Creating Sustainable Beliefs

The moment you start to question an existing belief, you start to weaken it. When you find that it has no root, or that its root is in situations that are no longer relevant to your journey, it loses its strength. Know when it is time to disassemble it completely and create new beliefs, if it is not relevant to your success.

We all have stories that we tell ourselves and others, about why we don't do what we are supposed to do for healthy living.

We tell the story so many times that we start to believe it. We blame our *situation, our time, the events we partake in, genetics, life's circumstances, etc.* We tell these stories so we don't have to try to lose the weight, or to excuse the habits we revert back to when we try and fail.

It's time to attack these stories and *rewrite* them. Take responsibility for your choices and behaviours; focus on the future rather than the past. Tell yourself, *Yes, I am limited by the stories that I tell myself why I cannot change my life. I, and only I, can rewrite these stories and refuse to let anyone else hold the pencil or pen to my story.*

Reframe your story for your genetics by repeating this one; I had to: *Yes, my genes determine some of the ways my body functions, but if I am overweight, I can lose it.* Redefine the story that you keep telling yourself. Replace *I'm too busy* with *yes I am busy, despite that, I can make quick and healthy meals at home, or cook ahead of time, to save me time in the future. I can order healthy foods when I eat out. It doesn't take time to eat healthy, it gives me time, it gives me quality over a lifetime.*

Reclaim your childhood by saying: *Although it was someone else who taught me to eat this way when I was young, it is now my responsibility to teach myself to eat the right foods, at the right time and in the right portions, to accomplish the goals I desire.* The more limiting stories you rewrite that you keep telling yourself, the less you will be held back by these beliefs.

Every new idea is limiting the first time you think or hear it. When you say to yourself, "This time I am going to change my life," it is only natural to have several limiting thoughts immediately follow. Believe in the truth and the truth is, if you are overweight or living an unhealthy lifestyle, YOU CAN change it.

> *One of the quickest ways to change, is to change the way you define yourself.*

Take time each day to reinforce new ideas (review the section on focus, and the *Hour of Power*). This is a time of empowerment where you expose yourself to positive and supportive messages, by taking the time to examine your victories and charting specific goals for the future. This is where you let go of the negative words of others and focus on your new beliefs and expectations. Use your visions, combined with your expectations, so that you begin to expect the vision to come true.

This may sound easy, but you may spend a great deal of time moving between the new stories and the old. You may struggle and exhaust great effort to effectively destroy the power of the old beliefs. This investment will be well spent, because in time, you will be able to question the old limiting beliefs enough to eventually weaken and break them.

What you are really doing is weakening your old *mindset* and developing a new one. You are undoing years of conditioning to start anew with a fresh learning experience. This is the true work of changing your *mindset* – what this book is all about.

Develop new beliefs that support you. All personal breakthroughs begin with a change in our beliefs. Successful people absolutely believe that they have the ability to succeed. Believe it is possible and you will do everything necessary to achieve the results you want. Believe that success will happen, since this time you are making the change from the inside out.

If you assume something is possible, then you will do the things necessary to reach your goal. If you believe something is impossible, you will not do what is necessary and you will not produce the desired results. Whatever you repeat often enough, becomes a new belief. The choice of what you believe is up to you.

Strengthening New Useful Beliefs

The only way to really make your new beliefs stick is to start the work. Do the new things you have chosen to do and do them frequently. Nothing helps reinforce new beliefs like the progress we make with them. Each little victory adds another stone to the foundation of your new belief system. As you accumulate these victories, you build a strong foundation that, with time, becomes as fundamental to your behaviours as the old ones were.

You must also understand what stands in your way of achieving your goals. Ask yourself what you need to believe to be able to achieve what you want. Identify, one at a time, the old beliefs and expectations that block your success. Analyze them, break them down, and replace them. Start new actions that will validate your new beliefs. Do this again and again, changing one unhelpful belief at a time when you identify them.

> To illustrate, do you really believe that you can maintain a healthy eating regimen long-term? Some people find it easy to start a new diet; they are so accustomed to the ritual of trying something new and being hopeful that they will lose weight immediately. However, the idea of maintaining a healthy eating regimen for life and not a *lose weight quick* diet, scares them tremendously.

> They quickly point to the past failures and the fact that they have never been able to keep the weight off long-term. Try to break down these beliefs. You may also want to seek the help of a health coach or dietitian and be candid about how you feel. Let him or her assist you with a sustainable eating and exercise regimen that is livable for you. You may also need to enlist the services of a psychologist or mental health therapist, if there are emotional issues or past

traumas that have produced self-deprecating, limiting beliefs.

Remember, you are the only one who can identify what beliefs are keeping you from your goals. Likewise, you are the only one who can change these blocks. Others may try to hold you back out of concern that you are making a mistake. Know that they mean well, but also remind yourself that you know best what changes are needed for your success.

Remember to keep all changes, great and small, realistic and livable. Making a sudden, extreme change can be difficult to deal with. The smallest changes are often the most effective. I had a client who believed that she would have to be hungry to lose weight. In fact, she gained this belief from a professional who told her that it was the only way to successfully lose weight. Of course, she was not willing to live with a constant feeling of hunger! Who would?

When she came to me, I helped her see that this belief was completely false. We identified foods that were healthy and how eating them at the right time and in the right portion size would keep her full, satisfied and closer to her weight loss goal every day. With her new nutrition plan in hand, she realized that she was eating a lot healthier and a lot more then she ever expected while still losing weight without feeling hungry. In fact, she would tell me all the time that the plan included so much food that she couldn't finish it all most days. Soon, she was well on the way to losing all the extra weight she wanted

– just that one belief about hunger had held her back for so many years!

Another client believed that she would not be able to sustain a healthy diet because her family was not practicing it with her. She didn't want to do it alone and felt her new changes would be awkward for her family and she wouldn't get any support. Added to that was the effort it would take to make different meals for her and the rest of the family.

After we worked through these limiting beliefs, she realized that she indeed had options that would not make her life as difficult as she anticipated. As she accepted the new belief that she could eat healthy on her own and without creating awkward situations, she believed that she could create the life she wanted and she did. Also, she found out over time, that her family loved eating the way she was and wanted to join her new lifestyle. This allowed everyone to benefit from her efforts.

When you get the idea that you are going to change your life, and add emotion to it, there is going to be a ping pong battle in your head. Your old, controlling beliefs resurface; all the things you were taught to believe and accept things the way they are. Beliefs that it will not work this time, just like all the others, and that you can't do it so why try.

Your old *mindset* will always tell you what you cannot do when you try something new. If you really analyze most of your disempowering beliefs, they are not sound and have no foundation. They are baseless lies; stories that we tell ourselves that just are not true. You will only get as far as your beliefs will let you. Change your *mindset,* believe in yourself and go for it.

3. Your Purpose: Your "Why"

The third and final pillar of motivation is your why. You can have a vision and modify your beliefs, but you need to ask yourself, *Why am I doing this*?

> *As your vision is your map, and your beliefs are your guide, your "why" is the fuel to push you through your journey.*

The most important thing in creating a motivated *mindset* is knowing why you want to do this. *Why do you want to change your life? What is your purpose? Why is it worth it to you?*

At this point, it doesn't matter what your answer is, what matters is how strong and powerful it is to you. You may want to look leaner, become a body builder, or be as healthy as you can. You may want to avoid certain health risks, get off of certain medication, or get rid of health problems that you have. You may want to improve your relationships or join an activity that you presently cannot. You may want to get healthy for your children and/or grandchildren, or travel and be fit enough to do so.

DOUBTFUL DIETING TO LASTING LIFESTYLE CHANGE

Everyone has a why. It's the value and importance you make your why that will determine your life change.

Everyone has a why. We are told that we need to have a why, that people fail because they don't have a why. So why do people fail even if they know their why? The reason is that they don't have a high enough value on their why. Your why will always be there, but when you hit the "lows" of your journey it's the value or the importance you put on your why that will push you through. If it is of high enough value to you. The higher you can keep that value and importance on your why, and you add a belief and vision to support it, will cause you to take constant actions towards your goals.

Why is it that only a few people will change that actually want to change, even if they all have a reason to change? The few that change have a higher level of importance and value on why they need to change. How do you make something important, you emotionalize it.

There is power in your "why." My father's *why* was inspired by having a heart attack. After discovering that smoking was one of the major causes of his heart attack, his why was that he didn't want to die. Despite being a smoker for almost 50 years and unsuccessfully trying to quit for about 10 of those years, he quit smoking that day and has never looked back. He did not want to go through another attack, after being blessed to survive the first one. Although that is a very powerful "why," some may not survive the extreme of such a health crisis.

The exact reason is not as important as the value of that reason to you. A truly valuable purpose will help you on days when the transitional costs seem too much. It will pull you back from the temptation to give up on a day when you can't trust your results. Your *why* equals power.

Your "why" will always come before your "how."

The *how* of your life change always follows the *why*. Having a powerful and irresistible *why* will provide you with the necessary *how* to do it. In other words, if you have big enough reasons to do something, you will figure out how to do it. Also, no matter what diet and exercise plan you follow, if you have strong enough reasons to follow it, you will find a way to succeed.

It is easy to slip back into old habits and patterns, but strong reasons to continue on your path will bolster your resolve when it starts to falter. If you have not followed through on your goal to lose weight before, it is because you did not have strong enough reasons to do so. Your reasons need to be personal and intimate in order to be your driving force.

There are a hundred of reasons "why not," but it only takes

one great reason why.

Every one of my client's success stories belonged to someone who had a powerful motive to change. If your reasons for change is strong enough, you will change. Keep asking yourself *why* and build a compelling list of reasons that mean the world to you to follow it through. Make a list of at least five reasons, then keep going and make as long as a list as you can. Continually ask yourself "why" followed by a hard look at the list. The one that is the deepest and closest to you will prevail and it is usually the last one on the list. The deeper you go, usually the deeper the emotional connection. If you allow yourself to be driven by this purpose, you are sure to be motivated to achieve success.

Your daughter's upcoming wedding may inspire you to lose weight for your public appearance, but what will motivate you to keep the weight off? After the event is over, it will be easy to revert to old habits if that was the only reason why you lost weight.

However, learning that your first grandchild is on the way, may inspire a life change. If you experienced a parent that died prematurely as a result of weight related health issues, you definitely don't want to follow in their footsteps. Your first grandchild might be the motivation needed to make the necessary changes so you will stand a fighting chance of living long enough to see him or her get married.

Changing Purposes

For a lot of people, the *why* that drives them initially may change over time. This is why it's a good idea to re-evaluate your why periodically. One clue to a change in your goals is that you start to lose a sense of purpose.

What is your purpose? What do you propose to do about it? This is not to be confused with feeling overwhelmed or tired. A loss of purpose is not when you question whether you want a goal you have chosen; it is when you know that you want it but are unable to articulate the reasons for wanting it.

I had a client whose initial reason for losing weight was *she wanted to be healthy*. This reason was enough to drive her efforts for most of her weight loss journey. But as she came close to her goal weight, she started sensing a change of purpose. Losing weight and being healthy by itself was no longer enough for her.

During her journey, her experiences had helped her feel youthful, energetic and excited. She was feeling the power of youth through her new found fitness. She was over 75 years old and retired; she would tell me about how she would go to these *tea gatherings* with her friends. The tea always included unhealthy foods with it.

One day, as she was sitting at a table for one of these gatherings, she noticed how everyone of her friends around her was suffering from some kind of health issue – diabetes, high blood pressure, obesity, needed a hip replacement, etc. When we reevaluated her *why*, she realized that her new purpose was to keep feeling this youthful energy and stay as healthy as she could, while keeping off all the weight she lost. She was full of energy and had no health problems and that's how she wanted to stay. In her words, she "wanted to die young at an old age."

You may also find that your own purpose is modified by, or evolves through, your experiences. This is a good thing; it means that your experiences have allowed you to find something that is valuable to you and this new experience is something that you have come to deeply desire.

For those of you who do not experience any change in your purpose, it simply means that your initial *why* was the most powerful desire you had or needed for this journey. You may or may not find a new purpose later in life, but for today, your *why* is the most powerful one, and it is all you need.

Your real driving force is not your 'will' power; it's your 'why' power!

Willpower only lasts for so long, and as it may be great to get you started; it's your *why-power* that keeps you going. For example, your willpower may initially get you to start going to the gym, but your "*why-power*" will keep you going to the gym.

Your *why* is your reason(s), your fuel. It's what builds your determination. You need strong enough reasons to make the trip through this journey.

Final Words

The ignition to sustained motivation starts with your vision of who you are and who you want to become. You have to adopt a body image that will inspire you and your efforts. This will give you the inspiration needed to help define the direction and path of your journey. This is your map to where you are going.

You also have to expect that this change will happen for you, to believe in yourself. You will need to develop a belief that you can truly achieve your vision. Without the belief in your own abilities, you will find yourself without the conviction needed to complete the journey. When you are assured that you can reach your goals and realize your vision, you will have created the guidance system that will take you there. Your vision is your map, your beliefs are your guide; you have to believe you can and you will.

Finally, to keep you going on the worst days, you need to know your purpose or your *why*. Your *why* is your fuel; knowing the deepest and truest reasons why you are taking the required efforts, will help you overcome your desire to quit and fill you with a sense of purpose that will lead you to success.

When you truly own all these three, you will find that you have transformed your hesitant and skeptical *mindset* to a motivated one. Your journey is now well underway; you will start to fight non-supportive emotions with these empowering emotions. Remember, your vision is your map; it gives you inspiration to move forward. Your beliefs are your guide; when you believe, you have hope and when you have hope, you have options to move you forward.

Your *why* is your reasons, your fuel; it builds your determination. You need to have strong enough reasons to make the trip. When you are inspired, have hope and determination, this will give you the sustained motivation to forge ahead.

Action Steps:

Find your vision: Take a piece of paper and write down your vision for your life; make it as clear as possible. Describe every little aspect that you want to achieve. *How do you feel? What do you look like body wise, health wise, vitality wise, etc.? Describe the things that you will be able to do, the clothes you will be able to wear.* Describe, while using all five senses, as much as you can. The clearer your vision, the more motivated you will be to get there. Find photographs of yourself at your goal weight or those of people whose fitness/body/lifestyle you idolize; use these pictures to strengthen your image of yourself. Use a favourite piece of clothing that will fit you when you reach your goal to motivate you. If your final goal involves a lot of weight loss, you may want to visualize yourself at various stages along the way to help you reach each small goal. If you have 100 lbs. to lose, vision yourself with 10 lbs. off; then, when you get there, vision another 10 lb. loss.

Build beliefs and expectations: Start by identifying limiting beliefs that you may hold. Examine each, one by one, and see where its roots may be. Recognize that some beliefs will be baseless; others have roots in experiences that are no longer relevant to your journey. Attack those beliefs that don't support you, while building an alternate belief based on you fulfilling your goals. Use your efforts and victories to strengthen these beliefs. Keep a diary with these beliefs listed; add each strengthening event to the list, so that you can read these entries and motivate yourself.

Find purpose: Make a list of at least five reasons why you want to achieve the goals that you set for yourself. Dig deep. If you think there are more reasons, add them as well as many as you possibly can. Keep asking the question, *why?* Use these reasons to motivate you; continue making a list and reading it daily. Periodically, re-examine your purpose and see if you have found new reasons that motivate you. Keep the priority of your list of reasons flexible and use the most powerful ones to motivate you as this list shifts.

Always take time periodically to re-evaluate and renew your vision, beliefs and your *why*.

You Only Get Results By Taking Action

#4. The Principles Of Taking Action For A Lifestyle Change

By now you have made the commitment to change and you are focused and have learned what you will have to do to motivate yourself. You know how to draw on your innermost desires and put yourself into an action *mindset*. But all of this means nothing if you don't take action.

Until you take action, the idea you have is just that – an idea, a thought and a dream. Although envisioning your goal and pushing yourself to believe in it may be a huge step, the vision will die unless you feed it with the results produced by action. You might have the deepest, greatest *why* for what you must do, but nothing actually changes until you take action.

As you start to make an effort, you will start to see results. These results will take you closer to your goal weight and ideal fitness. Each change you see will also feed your new *mindset* and strengthen your new attitudes, beliefs, and new comfort zone. With consistent action, you will soon find that you have adapted to your new lifestyle and are a happier, fitter and healthier version of yourself.

Unfortunately, there is no shortcut to success produced by consistent action. It takes time, dedication, and persistence. Jim Rohm said, and I agree with him, that the *formula for success ... is a few simple disciplines practiced every day. Then you start a whole new process, a whole new life.*

Well, the opposite is also true: *the formula for failure is a few errors in judgment repeated every day.* Every little bit adds up until, a few years later, you can't recognize yourself. But the reverse is also true – a few right choices every day lead to consistent success. A new exercise routine, healthier food and appropriate portion sizes, with time, lead to a slimmer, healthier, and happier you.

The 80 – 20 Rule

Does your required life change feel like a lot of pressure to do the right thing each time, every time? Let me simplify it for you. You don't have to do something 100 percent correct, 100 percent of the time: this is a lifestyle change, not a diet. What you have to aim for is 80 percent, which means that you can

DOUBTFUL DIETING TO LASTING LIFESTYLE CHANGE

indulge once and a while; you have to manage how often *once in a while* occurs.

I tell my clients to try to *choose* these occasions by planning ahead and planning the days around it so they don't get too off track. Eating one *off meal* won't hurt you, but if you eat it this way often, it will add inches to your waist and put you on the reverse track to success. It's not the "treats" that matter, it's if these "treats" become habits which is where the problem lies. (It's about what you do *most* of the time, not some of the time.) A lot of "dieters" get caught up in the slip ups that happen some of the time, which causes them to derail off course.

Consistency is what matters, so by contrast, eating a few healthy meals doesn't count. You have to eat these healthy foods most of the time, so that you can lose excess weight and still enjoy your favourite treats occasionally. With time, you will find new, healthier foods that you enjoy and a decreased desire for the 20 percent allotment for treats.

I find that, with most of my clients, this percentage decreases on a weekly basis. Why? Because you are what you eat, or in better words, you feel what you eat. When you start eating healthy consistently, every day you feel great and you really notice when you have overindulged in unhealthy foods. You can feel the difference.

When you eat something unhealthy, like a big bag of chips right before bedtime, you wake up drowsy and tired. I tell my clients that they are having a "food hangover," whenever they feel different after eating an unhealthy choice. When you eat clean, you feel clean; when you eat healthy you feel healthy.

I had a client come in for the first time and I said, *you are what you eat.* He looked at me and said, *well, I currently eat a lot of fast food; does that make me fast, cheap, and easy?* I told him that's not what I was saying, but he had a good point.

You cannot be a perfectionist when it comes to a lifestyle change. Yes, strive for perfection, but know that it is unattainable for the rest of your life. Things are going to happen that you don't expect; the key is that you get up and get back on track right away. This buffer of 20 percent may be very important to you for this reason, especially on the days when you have low motivation.

Remember, treat your daily goals like a rubber band. On a day when you can stretch and push yourself, do more. Meet more process goals and try to exceed them. But on days when you are ready to give up, give yourself some leeway; do just the smallest, most basic of your daily goals. Whatever you do, just keep moving forward in some capacity.

Habits

Motivation is what gets you started, but it's habit that gets you there.

DOUBTFUL DIETING TO LASTING LIFESTYLE CHANGE

I am often asked, *what is the secret to success?* I say, *success is found in your daily routine, your habits.* What are you consistently doing, every day? You become who you want to become by your daily habits.

You want to become healthier? Do something that increases your health every day. You want to lose weight? Create daily habits that will get you closer to where you need to be. These are choices, decisions and disciplines, we set up.

In order to achieve a new life for yourself, you have to perform at a different level. In other words, you cannot solve your weight problem, or achieve your goals, at the same level you are today. You have to become excellent at some new habits.

The wonderful thing is, all habits are learn-able. You can learn the skills necessary for success and find a way to incorporate them into your daily routine. *Wouldn't it be great if you could take a pill, do one sit up, or eat an apple and get into the best shape of your life?* It doesn't work that way; it takes persistence, consistency and time to develop new healthy habits that will take you there.

90 to 95 percent of what we do is out of habit. Everyone has habits that may not serve them well; the trick is to have an awareness of what is holding you back and identify some of the habits you need to develop to get the results you want.

Our brains are committed to being extraordinarily efficient in order to run our lives smoothly. If we had to think consciously about every single thing, it would become impossible for us to function. Thus, the brain makes us take shortcuts for all the situations that it possibly can, to reduce the amount of conscious processing that it has to do.

Anything we do on a regular basis becomes a habit as a way to reduce thinking about it. The brain doesn't differentiate between what's a good habit and what's bad. It doesn't matter what that action is – it could be smoking after supper or going for a walk after supper. If you do it often enough, the brain will create a shortcut for it and urge you to follow that habit.

You cannot just get rid of habits, you have to replace them. Habits fulfill a need. If you want to break unhelpful habits that you have, you must find new, healthy ones that fill the same need but produce the desired results. If you don't do this consciously, you may find another unhelpful habit replacing the first one.

It's like gardening: if you want to grow herbs, it's not enough to pull out the weeds; you have to plant the herbs and care for them too. Otherwise, your herbs will not grow to the best of their abilities and you will produce more weeds for you to tackle. You have to consciously and deliberately replace an unhealthy habit with a healthy one, or you may end up magnifying the problem.

So how do I replace these bad habits, you ask? The first thing to do is identify just one unhelpful habit that you have – something that is holding you back from your goal. Write it down and then write its polar opposite, something that you can confidently exchange it with.

For example, are you in the habit of eating unhealthy foods for your unpleasant emotions? First, identify that you do that. Next, identify the need emotional eating fills. What emotion is it used for? Then choose a healthy alternative, like going for a walk or a hot bubble bath, to get you away from the kitchen. Alternately, add something healthy and comforting to your routine, so that the desire to eat something unhealthy is not triggered. Now practice this new choice each and every time the unpleasant emotion surfaces, until your healthy alternative becomes a habit. There will be days that this is easier to do than others; the key is to be consistent.

The most common question people ask me about forming new habits is, *How long will it take for the new behaviour to become a habit?* The answer varies from person to person; for some, a few months, for others it may take six months or a year. The difference depends on the strength of the old habit, how deeply rooted it is and the effectiveness of the new one. An individual's preferences and personality also play a part.

Some people need a push to make an immediate change – like my father, who tried unsuccessfully to quit smoking many times before having a heart attack. The heart attack was strong enough motivation and he quit completely, never to return. He had a strong enough *why* that he thought that he will die if he continues.

But, for the most, we don't experience such dramatic moments to trigger change; we must make them consciously. We have to be persistent and follow through on the new choice until it becomes a habit. Give yourself 30 days of consistent practice for any habit to take place. Do the same thing for 30 days – everyday give yourself that initial momentum. If you miss or skip a day, simply start the 30-day cycle all over again; never give up on the 30 days. Once you have completed 30 consistent days and you feel confident that you have worked this new habit into your routine, start another new healthy habit (while maintaining the previous one), for the next 30 days. Repeat.

> *Unhealthy habits are easy to form, but hard to live with. Healthy habits are hard to form but easy to live with.*

Your new self is dependent on the new habits that you choose today. Replace unhelpful habits with healthier ones. Slowly, you will see yourself change physically because your automatic desires have changed internally. The more unhealthy habits you identify and replace, the faster you will see yourself moving toward your goals. After all, so much of what we do is because of our habits.

> *Know the difference between a treat and a habit.*

This is an important difference. A treat is something that we give ourselves on occasion, maybe to pamper ourselves or when we have had a particularly crazy day. It's nice but optional. But when the treat happens more and more frequently, it quickly morphs into a habit that we cannot function without. Remember, our brains are particularly good at forming habits. So when any unhealthy behaviour becomes a frequent occurrence, it can easily become a habit. Sometimes without noticing, underneath our radar, this unhealthy behaviour happens more and more frequent, then you have a habit, and the habit has you.

Triggers

If all it takes for a new habit to form is persistent activity, why are some old habits so hard to break away from? It's because they are triggered. A trigger is *any situation or experience that reminds us to follow through on a habit*. When two things occur together often enough, the occurrence of one triggers our desire for the other. For example, eating popcorn at the movies. Many of us naturally associate going to the movies with eating popcorn and other "movie treats." Despite what meal we had before or during the movie, most of us will add popcorn to our movie ticket purchase.

If we try to change our habits, without making any changes in the environment around us, we find that our old habits are notoriously hard to do away with. This is because they are still being triggered by our surrounding things and situations.

It is our job to identify these triggers that are unhelpful to us, and change the situation or substitute an effective, healthy response to the trigger. First, you have to develop an awareness of what are the triggers and associated routine that you are engaged in. The more changes you make, the more healthy habits you will form. The more healthy habits you have, the more you will feel the push to form other healthy habits which are related to your existing healthy habits.

Habits have buddies: like begets like.

You can use triggers to your advantage. If your current naturally occurring triggers can activate your unhealthy habits, you can create naturally occurring triggers that activate your healthy habits. It all starts with a trigger.

Give yourself reminders to do the healthy things. Keep healthy food where you can see it and unhealthy ones hidden. Keep your exercise clothes next to your bed to trigger you to take a morning walk. Put up post-it's or use an app to remind you to do an exercise or some stretches before work, at your desk. Leave a bottle of water on your desk so you will be reminded to drink water regularly. There are many simple phone applications that can help you trigger the helpful habits that you want to cultivate. Find and use whatever tools you need to trigger the habits you want to form.

Food Triggers

A uniquely complex trigger is one that makes us eat certain foods. This trigger is a situation that stimulates you to eat, which could be a helpful response or non-helpful to achieving your goals. Most of us have a lot of food triggers – like being in a coffee shop may trigger eating something sweet or crunchy with our coffee simply because we see it. Indulging in this matter, over time, may produce a habit of always having something sweet and/or crunchy with your coffee.

A huge part of your success will depend on whether you are able to identify and respond to your unhealthy food triggers. Remember that these are often deep-seated, so you may have to change your environment to deactivate them. Some of the actions that can help change food triggers are:

Modify your eating environment. Do you sit in front of a TV while eating your meals? This may make you unconscious to how much you are eating. Choose another seat.

Think differently about food. Teach yourself to like new, healthier options and cue eating them instead of unhealthy ones.

Deal with your emotions in a productive way. Emotions can be powerful triggers. Try to incorporate exercise, meditation or even deep breathing into your routine, to help balance out emotions and reduce their impact.

Make eating healthy a higher priority than pleasing others.

Solve the problems, don't distract with food.

Dr. Judith Beck describes in her book, The Beck Solution, the various triggers that can make us eat. It could be seeing or smelling food; real hunger or thirst; an emotional or mental trigger; reading about food, recalling something you enjoyed eating or a social trigger – like watching someone eat or trying to fit in by eating what everyone else is eating. Dr. Beck goes on to say that the only way to effectively respond to these triggers is to first identify that a food trigger exists. Once you are consciously aware of what is happening, you can create a substitute response that is healthier. It will not be easy, but because you are doing it consciously, you know what has to be done. Make the substitution often enough and you will create a new pairing of your trigger to a healthy response.

Everyone has triggers; the key is knowing what to do when you are triggered. First, you have to recognize or be aware of the people, emotions, situations, environments, and any other triggers for unhealthy eating. Then you must retrain your mind to behave a different way other than using food or self-sabotaging habits. You do this by consistently taking action on your new healthy ways, by creating new triggers/cues that will prompt you to take these new actions until these actions become habits. A good example would be if you wanted to start walking or an exercising routine every morning when you get up. A way to cue this trigger would be to place your walking/workout gear (clothes, sneakers, etc.) right by your bed the night before, and as soon as you wake up put them on.

This is a great way to trigger yourself to start this new routine in the mornings.

Typically, people create a cycle, I call it the *typical diet cycle*. A person starts their new diet, but then a trigger happens for an unhealthy response. The person behaves the way they used to behave; they feel guilty about it which creates more stress, which creates more feelings of shame and guilt. This causes an emotion that the dieter thinks about, then typically acts on this emotion by sabotaging his or her success. More distress follows and then increases when their action(s) works against their diet. This starts a vicious and often self-defeating cycle.

Yes, when you start to take action, you need a healthy plan to follow, but you have to learn how to recognize triggers that affect your goals. By knowing what your triggers are, you can reset your weight set point and eliminate your destructive patterns. Set yourself up to win by providing yourself with triggers that cue a new routine that promotes new actions that will feed into your success.

Actions To Take

Yes, you need the right *mindset* to succeed, but you also need to have the right strategies; without them, no matter how hard you try, you will not get the desired results. No matter how far you run east, you won't see the sunset. As I mentioned earlier, this is a *how to* vs. a *what to do* book. I will not be giving you a meal or exercise plan with this book. I will give you the necessary strategies you have to take to make a successful life change no matter what health plan you choose to follow, versus going on just another short-term diet.

Now that we know how habits are formed and how to respond to triggers, let's focus on the actual actions that you can start doing today to make effective changes.

Study

If you want to be fit, you first have to study how to become fit. You have to study what to do to become fit, what to do for exercise and what to eat, etc. If you want to become healthier, you have to study how to become the healthiest version of yourself.

Take some time and collect information about diets, nutrition, portion sizes, exercise routines, and recipes that are healthy and tasty. Study cooking, preparation, and other healthy options that you can incorporate into your lifestyle. There is an abundance of information out there; just have patience in finding the ones that work for you.

Search the internet, buy a book or get a CD/DVD; find plans that work for you. Also pay attention to information that explains how some things are not good for you; study the positive and negative. Sometimes you may find a lot of options and become confused about what you should choose. Ask someone you trust. You may even want to invest in yourself with a dietitian or nutritionist, a food coach, or a personal trainer, and study the information from them.

When studying what to do, always ask yourself two questions: *Is this healthy to the best of my knowledge? Is this livable for me?* Study other people; study someone who had the same struggles as you and turned their life around. What did they do to change their life? Success leaves clues; failures leave footprints. If someone is struggling and has never succeeded in any change, study what they are doing and don't do it.

> *You may not be able to do all that you find out, but find out all you can do.*

Learn

When you start collecting the information, don't just sit there. Learn from it and understand how what you are learning applies to your own circumstances. Learning and understanding the impact of your choices will help you make decisions that are helpful for your long-term health goals. Let your decisions be informed and guided by facts rather than whims and informal advice. If necessary, take a professional's help in the process of making choices.

> *Don't let all your learning turn to knowledge; you won't get anywhere. Your learning must turn into action.*

Learn from what you study, then take action. Try and learn – at any moment of a decision, the best thing you can do is the right thing. The next best thing is the wrong thing; the worst thing you can do is nothing. If you have a great week, learn from it; what did you do to make it a great week? If you have a bad week, learn from it; what happened to make it a bad week?

Try and learn, try and learn, try and learn. But don't let all your studying and learning lead to knowledge; knowledge alone will not produce results. You must take what you learn and act on it; always take action.

First, learn from your own experiences; experiences provide a rich source of information. You can learn a lot about what has been helpful, and what has not, by observing the impact of your past choices. What worked for you in the past and what didn't? Why couldn't you make a lifestyle change from what you did before? How can you change that? Something that works for another person may not work for your life's circumstances.

Don't forget to consider your failures in the process. Remember that every failure tells you something about what doesn't work for you. Knowing what doesn't work for you, allows you to quickly eliminate that choice from your options. Try not to think of it as a failure; rather, think of it as an unsuccessful experiment or lesson learned, that has taken you a step closer to finding the best options.

You can also learn from the experiences of others, as long as you don't make comparisons to your past efforts. Look at the choices made by friends, family or even role models, who had the extra weight but became fit. Sometimes, seeing what helped others can inspire you to try a technique you had not thought of. Model them while thinking of your own life and circumstances.

Remember to learn from people who made lasting healthy changes to the way they lived; not people who just went on a crash diet. Also remember to ask yourself if their choices are livable for you or whether you should try something else. Everyone has different circumstances; what worked for someone from a very different background and situation, may not work the same way for you. Also, learn from the mistakes of others. See how unhelpful choices affected them and make a mental note to avoid the same pitfalls.

> ***Successful people constantly learn and grow; unsuccessful people think they already know.***

Start A Nutrition Program

As I stated at the onset of this journey, this book can accompany any reasonable program that is healthy and livable. So I won't tell you what to eat or what to avoid. Different healthy diets work for different people, depending on their needs, overall health, social, and religious choices, etc. You can find many good nutrition plans online, in books or from your health professional. There is no lack of information out there on what to eat or how to exercise. See what works best for you, and start doing it.

Having a degree in Nutrition and also a Personal Trainer Specialist, I know what works for most people and what doesn't; what is healthy and what is not for most, but it doesn't matter unless you first follow the fundamentals and principles in this book. You may choose from any plans that you think will work the best for you, as long as it fulfills two criteria: 1) it is healthy, to the best of your knowledge and 2) it is livable for you. If you are not sure, please ask a professional or someone you trust.

If you are taking the advice of a professional, he or she can help you choose foods that will fit into your unique circumstances. However, be weary of the *quick fixes*. There are a number of diets that help you lose weight quickly, but I'm in the business of helping you get rid of your weight long-term, not just temporarily. *Quick fix* diets are typically not livable on a regular basis and are sometimes unhealthy. The moment you stop the diet, you regain all the weight you lost, sometimes even more. Stop focusing on how quickly you can lose weight; think of how you can change to get rid of the excess weight for good. What actions can you make now and continue forever? Will your chosen plan allow that?

Change is hard, especially in regards to food; often, any change feels unlivable. If you are feeling overwhelmed, make individual changes until you incorporate them into your everyday life. Start with a simple one – for example, drinking more water. Slowly add this to your repertoire of healthy choices. Ask yourself, *Can I live with this choice long term – at least 80 percent of the time?* Remember, that includes healthy choices and all the other benefits associated with it.

Healthy living is something positive that can add health, pleasure and energy to your life. Everybody has their own way of defining and living this. Find your own golden meaning and you will find food becoming a positive experience in your life in every way. You must find a nutrition plan that reflects this for you.

Exercising/Physical Activity

We all know that physical activity helps us burn the energy that we get through food. We also know that we need physical activity, not only to help lose excess weight and become fit, but also to improve our overall health. Many people believe that one has to run marathons or spend hours a day in the gym to lose weight. This is definitely not the case.

What is really necessary is to get moving and do what you can. Do something, anything, and build momentum. I always recommend that people start with something that they like or enjoy, so that exercise becomes a habit.

The best exercise is anything that you do consistently, that makes you move and that pushes your boundaries of strength and endurance, a little at a time. The most important aspect of exercise is making it a routine. Doing something regularly has far more benefits than doing a lot occasionally.

If you are not doing anything right now, start small – a 15 minute walk three days a week is a great place to start. Or participate in a sport that you like that you can play regularly or join a beginner's fitness class. As this becomes comfortable, add in more time and more exercises that you can do daily. Remember to choose things that can fit into your lifestyle and that you enjoy doing, but still lead you to incremental steps towards your improved fitness.

The key in any fitness routine is to start.

Make sure you find ways to get yourself to show up to your new activities. Make a schedule and *keep it*. You may want to use a journal/workout log or a reminder that goes off at a particular time each day. Again, it's not what you do *some of the time*, but what you do *most of the time* that matters. Make regular activity a part of your life. Schedule it and make sure you get there. Like anything else that is for your health – a doctor's appointment or dentist – put in on your schedule and show up.

Remember, different activities suit different people. You can walk, jog, run, hike, lift weights, golf, ski, kayak, or play a sport.

DOUBTFUL DIETING TO LASTING LIFESTYLE CHANGE

You can do this competitively or casually; you can do it alone or as part of a group. You can spend money on a gym or you can do activities that are essentially free. None of these are important issues; what *IS* important is that you are active for some time each day.

Some of you may feel that you do not enjoy *any* activity. I can tell you this without a doubt – there is some activity out there that you can do and enjoy on a regular basis. The key is to find that one thing that works for you. If you want to get more active, get around people that are more active than you; it will eventually rub off on you.

You may want to get a walking buddy or join a group/class. These are fun options that will also keep you accountable. Some of you may want to hire a personal trainer who can help push you beyond your limits. When you become comfortable with one activity or one level, push onto the next level or another activity. Challenging your own fitness levels is the key to motivating yourself.

A lot of us look at the gym as a place of intimidation. We worry about how we will be judged and what others will think. They don't think; at least not about you. Trust me, people are more worried about their own workout in the gym and have no time or energy to judge you. Even if they do, they are not worth your time – you are. The important thing is that you start moving while constantly challenging and pushing yourself to become fitter and healthier. When you are in the gym, be there. It's not how much time you put into the gym, it's how much gym you put into the time. It's the quality not the quantity when it comes to your time in the gym and your exercise routine.

Balance For Joy

There is a reason you should choose an activity you enjoy. Findings from Cornell University Food and Brand Lab show that when people are involved in activities they dislike, they eat more as a way to compensate. They conducted a study where they led adults on a 2 km walk around a small lake. One group of people were told it was a scenic walk; the other group were told it was an exercise routine. The ones who thought they were forced to exercise, ate 35 percent more chocolate pudding later. Those who thought that they were being helped to enjoy themselves, felt less desire for the pudding.

Basically, when we are happy with our activity choices, we add to our positive emotions. But when we feel like we don't enjoy the activity, we make up for these negative emotions by eating more – and effectively sabotaging ourselves.

This brings me to another important point. No matter what activity you choose, you can never out exercise a bad diet. People often believe that if they exercise, they can eat whatever they want. Some believe that they can just spend more time at the gym to erase the effects of unhealthy eating habits. Nothing could be further from the truth.

From my educational background, and decades of client experience, I can assure you that there is no such thing as *exercising it off or away*. You have to eat healthy most of the time if you want to stay healthy. The right nutrients are needed not just for weight loss, but to maintain overall health and well-being. It is not wise to depend on diet or exercise alone as a means to stay fit. A combination of healthy eating and daily exercise is the formula for a long-term healthy lifestyle.

> *We do not stop playing because we grow old; we grow old because we stop playing!*
>
> **~Benjamin Franklin**

Hire A Coach

Hiring a coach can be one of your most valuable tools for your life change. In this world of doubters and naysayers, one of the best ways to stay on track is to have someone that you are accountable to. This someone can be a friend or a family member who understands the goals you have set. You could also hire a professional like myself – or a dietitian, nutritionist, food coach or a personal trainer.

Whatever your choice, go to someone who understands a healthy lifestyle and perhaps has gone through the journey themselves. You can also hire someone who has helped others go through the journey and has demonstrated results. If you choose to hire a professional, do your homework and decipher whether their ideas of a healthy lifestyle are in line with yours. Long term, you will only connect with those whom you share the same values with.

Having a coach who is on the same page as you means that they will share and understand your values and support the goals you set, helping you make the right choices to pursue those goals. At the same time, they are outside of you and will be able to hold you accountable, setting high standards for you to reach. Even on days when you are distracted, they will stay focused on your goals and will push you to do the same. You may be able to make excuses to yourself, but a committed coach will not, nor allow you to.

It is my belief, after my years of experience of being a coach and training coaches, that four things make a great coach:

Presence. A great coach is present or there. He or she allows no distractions; full attention is given to each client. At every session or visit, they are the main focus.

Connection. A great coach has the ability to connect to your values. When he or she finds a way to connect to your values, then and only then, will they be valuable to you. Identifying and connecting with your values, allows them to motivate you and find the right solutions for you.

Customized advice - the appropriate actions/solutions. A great coach will help you identify the right actions to take FOR YOU; the ones that give you the results you expect and desire.

Accountability and support. A great coach checks in and follows up with you regularly. They are there for you; rarely do you have to ask for their assistance.

You can't see the picture when you are in the frame. – Les Brown

You are the best judge of what you can and cannot do. But you are also easily influenced by your emotions and daily experiences. There will be days when you cannot separate your frustration from work or your workout time. On those days, you will think that you deserve a *day off*.

A coach is outside of your mind and will be able to see through the excuses that you make up. This will ensure that you at least meet your minimum goals, even on days when you are not motivated. Keep in mind, a coach isn't designed to be a dictator or insensitive to your struggles. I am not suggesting that they will be barbaric or a *you-will-workout-or-else* type leader. I am saying, however, that he or she will be your motivator and will not let you quit when you grow weary or tired.

I often find that clients may fall short because they think they know what is happening to them, but they don't know that they are stuck in their excuses or stories. This is where a coach comes in – or at least where I do with my clients. A good coach is a good detective; someone who is not you, yet is vested in your health. Your coach can help you separate your feelings and focus on your goals.

Because your coach keeps you on track and provides accountability and structure, you will be able to achieve consistent results. A good coach will also help you tweak your diet and exercise so that you are effectively challenged at all times but still properly nourished.

They understand your issues and concerns and are able to help you make good decisions. To ensure this, look for someone who shares your core values, is knowledgeable and personable, but also adaptable and capable of understanding any special circumstances that you may have.

Practice Mindfulness

One action step that needs to be taken – regardless of what program or plan that you may be following – is mindfulness. Mindfulness means that we are conscious and attentive to the things that are affecting us. When we are mindful, we understand how we are feeling and how we respond to different events. We also understand the impact of the different choices we make. We see ourselves making choices and seeing what effect it has on us. A mindful person receives more joy and satisfaction from each of his or her conscious choices, than someone who goes through the motions in a mindless manner.

Mindfulness is becoming more and more important for our physical as well as mental health. We live in a convenience based environment and are surrounded by choices that are easy and *convenient*, but often unhealthy. When we are not conscious of our choices, we are easily led by advertising tricks that make us choose these less helpful choices – simply because they are easy. So when you try to lose weight and live a healthier lifestyle, you are fighting your own emotions as well as the environment. It is easy to fall off track if you are not mindful.

There are so many instances of what happens when we are not mindful. According to studies in Dr. Brain Wansink's book "Mindless eating," we are 30 percent more likely to eat the first thing we see. So have "the good stuff" in the front of your kitchen shelves in the fridge and cupboards. Also, foods that are left out for you to see are eaten twice as fast.

Plate size. Plates today are, on average, over 20 percent larger then plates from the 60s. Weigh your food. Most of us are programmed to finish what's on our plate no matter how much is on there. The more in front of you, the more you eat.

Another study suggests that we are more likely to buy unhealthy foods if we shop on an empty stomach. Skipping meals can also sabotage your shopping. Even short-term food deprivation, even five hours, not only increases overall grocery shopping – these shoppers buy 18.6 percent more food – but also 44.8 percent higher calorie foods. The problem with these effects are that skipping a meal can cast a curse on your whole week, filling your pantry, fridge – and subsequently, belly – with more fattening foods.

One office research study showed that people eat more chocolate when they are given chocolates in a clear vs. opaque dish (because they can see the number of chocolates left). The difference was 71 percent more often than those given opaque dishes. Also, an office study revealed that you will eat less than half of these chocolates, if the dish is at least six feet away from where you sit.

On the other hand, food that comes in large packaging and large containers, encourages us to eat more (22 percent more), even if we don't like it. We also need to be mindful of our emotions while eating; people ate 28 to 55 percent more popcorn when watching a sad movie. People typically reach for more comfort foods when they are sad or tired, but reach for healthier options when they are happy. (People are 77 percent more likely to choose healthy foods when feeling happy).

The idea of being mindful is to understand how your environment influences your choices and to reduce this impact. In fact, you can even use these tricks to train your mind to eat better, by making healthy foods more accessible and by consciously responding to your negative moods.

But, by becoming mindful, you take back control in your own hands. You consciously choose what you eat and what you drink. You consciously choose what exercise to partake in. You consciously choose what message from your surroundings is useful and which ones need to be discarded.

Being mindful is a simple process but is rarely easy. We are not used to being aware of why we make certain choices; initially it is easy to revert to making mindless choices. Let it happen, but learn from that and apply your learning to the next time you find yourself in a similar situation.

Being mindful means understanding your own needs and what results you want. Know what people support your goal and mindfully include them in your life. Know what people hold you back, or are toxic to your success, and take a step away from them (even if just mentally).

You have to be mindful of food pushers, friendly saboteurs and food bullies. Use your new awareness to articulate your ideas and feelings to the people closest to you. When you are focused and clear headed, you will see that you do understand what you are doing and why, and you will feel more in control.

Meal Log

I don't care what plan you decide to follow, keeping a meal log is a great way to stay mindful of your new choices, habits and routine. I am a big believer in keeping a meal log/journal. A log or journal greatly increases your awareness of what you eat, when, how much and why you eat certain things. So often our minds trick us into thinking that we have eaten less than we actually have. The best practice is not to rely on your memory, but to write down everything you consume diligently when you are trying to create new healthy habits.

It only takes a couple minutes a day and is such a valuable tool when starting out on this journey. You need tools that will keep you accountable to yourself and the new habits you are developing. It has always been my policy in my clinic to tell my clients that, *if you bite it, write it. If you drink it, ink it.*

There are days when you break your rules and may not want to record the foods you have eaten. Being honest is the only way to understand what situations make you eat in unhelpful ways. Once you understand when these slip-ups occur, you will be better able to respond effectively. You can create an *if/then plan* – if this happens, then I will do this next time.

Look at "bad days" in the meal log as learning days. If you are honest about your reasons for eating, and if you use this information to make life changes, you will see that your unhealthy entries become fewer and fewer over time. If you can identify the triggers that invoke thoughts that lead you to eat in deconstructive ways, you can minimize your exposure or change your response to them.

Your meal log or journal will also help you to plan for problem areas or risky situations. You can make conscious choices of how to respond effectively to triggers that you anticipate; thus, you will be able to stick to your plan more effectively. Soon you will be logging more healthy foods frequently and you will have a meal log that reflects all the hard work you have put in. Keep all the information you put in your meal log/journal; this is valuable data, this serves as a record for future use. You can always look back at successes and problem areas that you changed. When someone asks you what is in your journal, you can respond, *this was the year that I changed my life and this is how I did it*.

Self-Awareness

Self-awareness is *a conscious knowledge of one's own character, feelings, motives and desires*. It is to know yourself deeply and *honestly*. It also means that you are aware of what you are good at and what you are not. Self-awareness means that you know your strengths and weaknesses and what areas you are most likely to fail.

To be self-aware means that you are able to harness your strengths and use them to make your chosen path easier to tread. It also means that you understand your failures and can reduce their impact on your goals, by accepting and working around them. The idea is not to become perfect, but to accept all that you are while being smart about your choices based on this knowledge.

For example, when I was counselling clients early in my career, I realized that my strength was that I made deep connections with my clients. I honed this strength so that it allowed my clients to be completely open with me. This way, I could further help them because they would tell me their true circumstances. This is why I was, and am, able to truly help them; they felt comfortable enough to tell me all the facts that I needed to help them.

Similarly, you will have strengths that help you stick to your goals – whether it is cooking, preparation, making effective reminders or something else. Use your strengths to propel you ahead. At the same time, be aware of your weaknesses – maybe your weakness *is not being able to say no to food you are offered*. Find a way around this: eat before you go out or agree to take only a tiny amount instead of the regular amount once and a while.

Final words

As you can see, there are many ways to take action and things you need to do for your life changing journey. You have to take the effort and deal with the initial discomfort, but you can also create a supportive environment that will enable you to get past this phase without giving up. The biggest step is to start and get your momentum going!

Know that you need to take action, but one step at a time. Be aware of your limits and push against them, but not so hard that you snap back into your comfort zone. Give it time and be consistent. Soon you will find that old habits are dying and new ones have started to replace them. Initially, don't worry about your final destination; it can be too overwhelming to think of how far you might have to go.

START, and build momentum by becoming consistent with the simplest new habits first. This will not only help you adopt the next habit, but will also build your confidence as you progress. Set daily goals for yourself and try to complete as many of these as you possibly can. Without realizing it, you will start inching towards that final goal.

Remember, it's not what you do some of the time, it's what you do most of the time that matters. It's what you do consistently; you will never change your life until you change something you do daily. Be specific about what you do, but also flexible in your approach. Mistakes will happen; accept that as part of the process, but leave room to revise the steps you plan out, especially if they turn out to be unsustainable or don't lead to the benefits you expected. Pay attention to what is working and what isn't; find substitutes when something isn't working.

Create mini goals; these are more realistic and you can plan effective steps for smaller goals. For example, your goal may be to lose 50 lbs. and you will find 20 ways to do it. But this is a big goal and it can be scary. First, focus on losing 10 lbs. and then another 10 lbs. As you keep losing weight in this manner, you will find that you have reached your goal of losing 50 lbs. The trick is to find the right actions and practice them daily. Remember to put most of your focus on your process goals and not so much on the end result. Find new healthy daily actions that you can easily incorporate into your life and work them.

The only way to succeed is to not give up. Join the estimated 5 percent of people who plan their lives intelligently and then reap the benefits for the rest of their lives.

Action Steps:

Habits: Make a list of the habits that are holding you back. Write down as many as you can think of. Now choose at least one of these habits and write down the exact opposite behaviour for it, or think of another healthy habit. Ask yourself, *is this a healthy action*? If it is, replace your old habit with the new one. Once you have adjusted to one changed habit, go back to your list and choose another unhealthy habit. Repeat the process with this one as well. Continue until you get through the entire list. It helps to start with the simple ones and then go onto the more deep-seated ones.

Triggers: Habits have triggers. Be a detective for yourself, find your triggers for your unhealthy habits and write them down. Become aware of how these triggers work for you. Find ways to deactivate old triggers by satisfying the underlying needs in a healthy manner. Make a list of what behaviours you want to instil and create triggers for the same. Activate the new triggers that will motivate you to practice your new, healthy actions.

Learning and choosing: Take half an hour each day to read up on health plans and healthy habits. This will also become part of your *hour of power*. Use the information you gather in this time to pick a health plan to follow. You can also do this by asking a health care provider.

First steps: Decide what is the #1 thing you can start doing right now. What could you start doing today, which if you did consistently, would have the most positive impact on your life? Remember to choose something doable and not a behaviour that is presently out of your reach. Also identify what is the #1 thing that you can stop doing, so that the absence of this behaviour has a positive impact in your life. When you have your answers, follow through immediately. You may find a number of answers to both questions, but pick one thing to do and do it.

Physical Activity: Find an activity that you enjoy and that is sustainable for you. Start small but do something every day. Remember that it should be something you enjoy, but pushes your fitness limits gradually. With time, increase the intensity of the activity or add in more activities that you enjoy. Work towards creating an exercise routine that is fun, and still challenging, by having a good mix of options.

Hour of power: As mention earlier, ensure that you eventually get in a minimum of half an hour of exercise per day. Also include half an hour of *innercise* – study and learning that will help you enhance your choices. This can include finding healthy food options, exploring exercise routines, reading, and recording recipes and listening to motivational, inspirational, informational messages, among other things. Remember to be mindful about your health for an hour each day; soon you will find that you are taking care of yourself consistently.

Hire a coach: Find someone who you trust and who understands your core principles. It could be a friend, family member or a professional. Tell them your goals and accept their help in deciding daily goals and rules. Ask them to hold you accountable. If this is a professional, ask them to review your actions to see where you can increase effectiveness.

Meal log: Keep a diary and write down everything you consume, how much and when. This includes what you eat, drink, recipes, portions and other similar things. If you can, at first, get a kitchen scale so you can measure what you are eating. This will help you identify ineffective portion sizes as well as serve healthy quantities. Make regular notations in your meal log and continue to do so until you feel you have mastered your nutrition.

Progressive steps: Change you "result goal" into a series of steps. Your result goal is just a problem you have to find an answer to. If it is to lose 50 lbs, ask yourself, *what can I do starting today to get rid of 50 lbs?* Write it down and list at least 15 answers to this question. Pick one to three of these answers and start acting on them today. Make daily goals that are doable and can help you start your journey. Once every couple of weeks, add to the intensity of your goals or add in another goal to your daily routine.

Self-awareness: Get the closest and most trusted people in your life to tell you what you are great at and not so great at. Identify strengths and weakness. Make a note of how each of your strengths can contribute to your goals. Also make a list of how each weakness can sabotage your goals and find ways to prevent this from happening. Take one strength and one weakness and apply what you learn about them to your daily routine.

Are You Getting The Results You Want?

#5. The Principles Of Getting Results For A Lifestyle Change

Nothing is more motivating than seeing progress.

Once we choose a plan of action and start working towards our goals, a lot of questions start to surface. *Are my actions leading to the results that I am looking for? Is the plan working for me?*

A lot of our desire to keep pushing forward is linked to visible results. We work better when we receive feedback and praise. We are more likely to visit a particular restaurant again if we receive good food and good service. We are more likely to stick to our plans if we see that the efforts we are taking are working. And this is the biggest challenge in sticking to our goals when we make lifestyle changes.

Being Patient

Many people give up on their goals or start to question the process when they see slower results. Sometimes they lose weight slower than they expected or wanted. Some weeks they see no change or worse, they see the scales go up.

At this point, the results are not giving them enough to want to continue and they start doubting themselves and the process. It's important to remember that the biggest difference between making a lifestyle change and going on a diet is the *approach*. If you are doing a juice cleanse for a week to lose the pounds fast, you will lose weight but these results are short lived; you will soon find yourself back at the starting point because you never made any long-term changes.

On the other hand, lifestyle changes are enduring changes in the way you think about and respond to food and exercise. This means that, while your initial results may be slow or fast, it takes you to change your *mindset* and set habits and learn new ones. The change that does occur will be permanent. Even the most gradual healthy changes start to add up and compound into a healthier you, not just a lighter you.

DOUBTFUL DIETING TO LASTING LIFESTYLE CHANGE

The doubts are understandable: if you don't see results, you don't know if you are on the right track. The best way to gauge this is to be patient and observe the progress, regardless of how slow. If you think that the changes are not adequate, observe your behaviours and choices across different situations, and then correct your course as necessary. Remember, in your actions you must be specific, but also flexible. With time, if you are not seeing the results you want, change your approach.

When you start making lifestyle changes, it can take some time to carry them out in all aspects of your life. Check if any particular area is giving you more trouble than others. For example, someone may easily make changes in their home life and in their workplace, but may have difficulty applying it to time with friends. Another person may be able to apply their chosen changes to home and friends, but may be unable to change their eating habits at lunches with colleagues.

If you find a crack in your armor, don't beat yourself up. Remember that each of the unhelpful eating habits have played a role in your life – from helping you connect with friends to finding common ground with colleagues and clients. For a new behaviour to take root, it has to fulfill the same needs as the old ones (maybe even improve on them). If this is not happening, it may be necessary to modify your new choices a little, to ensure that they work just as well as the old ones did, but in a healthier fashion.

Review and renew. What is working and what is not? Like I said, be committed, but be flexible in your approach. For the things that are not working, you can change your approach. How often do I have to change my approach? Until you succeed.

Plan, do and review; then repeat.

Flexibility is an essential virtue in this process; very rarely do people find the perfect fit to all their needs during the first attempt. Most often, we choose a new behaviour for its health benefits, but only then realize which needs the old one fulfilled. It is then necessary to modify the new behaviour, or replace it, so that it fits your health as well as other needs.

Take the example of a recovering drug addict or alcoholic. In recovery, clients are often encouraged to engage in healthy lifestyle choices as an alternative to their habits of addiction. Exercise may be their new addiction; one that they spend copious hours engaged in to fill their nervous energy and instil a sense of normalcy. However, anything done to the extreme, healthy or not, can be damaging. Exercising for four to five hours a day can create unhealthy, damaging results, although that wasn't the intent. The person in recovery would need to work with his or her advisor to find copings mechanism to address the real issues masked by this extreme behaviour.

Sometimes you need to change your approach; other times you may simply want to make the changes less intense. For some people, smaller changes may be best suited to starting lifestyle changes. But, as you progress, you may want to make even more effective course corrections. Especially when other people are involved, smaller, incremental steps can be more effective to get them slowly used to your new choices. These smaller steps are also easier for you to consistently follow through with, thus you are more likely to succeed.

> For example, expecting your family to be 100% in agreement to your new lifestyle regimen is a bit extreme for some. However, adding additional healthy options at meal times, as well as eating out once a week versus three times a week, may be received well.

Diets VS. Life Change: What To Expect

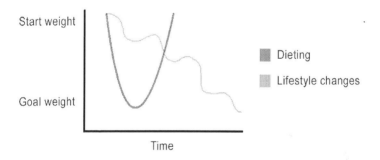

The above chart should help you understand what to expect from yourself. See how dieting can lead to drastic changes, quick results, but short-lived ones. On the other hand, the lifestyle changes that you are making may take a longer time to show an effect and will involve a series of ups and downs. But, over time, the body adjusts to the new, healthier habits and, as a consequence, to a new, lower weight set point.

Learning From Failure

Since we have established that lifestyle changes are a series of *ups* and *downs,* including weight fluctuations, let's take a moment and see what to do with the *downs*. When we do lose weight, it's a sign that the choices we have made are working for us. But when we notice the *ups*, the increases in weight, this is also a learning experience.

This is the time to be curious and not furious. It's easy to become upset when you don't see the results you want and just as easy to quit. But take a moment to understand which of your choices might have contributed to the increase. Be curious. Was it the party you attended where you decided to revert to old eating habits for a day? Was it a family event where you were overindulging in foods that you don't normally eat? Understand the situation. It is likely that each of these *ups* in your weight will help you find a new situation that needs your response. Always try to learn from your results; you can always find out why you are getting the results you are getting. There is always a reason; you just have to look for it, learn from it and apply it to your future actions.

Try to find solutions to the situations that are not helping you succeed. Did you fall off track? Then all you need to do is understand how this happened and how it affected you, then make choices that will help you avoid this in the future. Was it an external factor that you felt you were unable to control? This is a sign that you need to find effective solutions and plan for these occurrences.

Perhaps the choices you made did not work. You may need to modify them in some way. Remember that these are all learning experiences that will lead you to consistent and effective change. Even the short-term *failures* are valuable to you on this journey. Remember, failure leaves feedback; use it. Treat them as guideposts and course-correct by taking their feedback into consideration.

In making lifestyle choices, there is no such thing as failure, only feedback.

Be kind to yourself. Remember, life does happen, mistakes do happen; they are a natural part of the process. If you are making mistakes, it still means you are doing something. All you need to do now is to modify your approach and find a more effective response to the situations that are holding you back. Celebrate when you have a great week and learn when you don't.

A number of my clients tried to lose weight ten or more times before they came to me. They feel bad about it, but I always tell them that they should be proud that they haven't given up and are still trying. I tell them that the numerous attempts at a change are various lessons on what does not work for them. They should view these "attempts" as time savers or lessons in what not to do.

I help them to harness this information and use it to find out what does work for them and will lead to lasting changes. If you have had failures, use that as data; don't let it dishearten you. At least you now know what doesn't work for you; you can harness this information to propel you towards what does.

Keeping A Journal

This is also where meal logs can prove helpful. Our memories can conveniently lose information like portion sizes, frequency of eating, how much water we drank and snacks, especially if these are set habits. I've found that the really successful clients always maintain a meal log to ensure that they have the information they need. Every few weeks, they use this information to take stock of their journey and make changes and corrections as needed.

Meal logs can help you track what seemingly small habits may be sabotaging your own efforts; can help compare different phases of your journey as well as help you identify what choices are helpful and which ones are holding you back. I recommend you use one for at least a year. This is valuable data that your journal has in it; highlights of the year that you changed your life.

Strive For Progress, Not Perfection

Perhaps one of the most disheartening experiences for people trying to create long-term lifestyle changes is when they are overwhelmed by their own extreme expectations. Being a perfectionist and having absolute expectations is often a set up for failure, because there is no perfection when it comes to food habits. This is also the difference between creating a lifestyle change and going on a diet. A lot of people are perfect on their diet until it's over. We all know what happens after that.

It's great to have an ideal eating plan, but you need to accept early on that you cannot achieve perfect eating every day for the rest of your life. The trick is to draw up the ideal food and exercise routine and make these your habits (what you do most of the time). Try to achieve as much as you can, as often as you can; the more you can do on a particular day, the closer you are to your daily goal.

> *Perfection is the direction, not the destination.*

My favourite clients, (absolute sarcasm here), are the perfectionists. When it comes to eating, most perfectionists have an all or nothing approach. When they are on track, they are completely on; when they fall off (even just a little), they are completely off and it is hard to get them back on track right. The research shows that change happens more consistently, and lasts longer, when our goal is to get better and not perfect.

Celebrate each step closer to your daily and eventual goals, but don't lose heart on the days you don't reach your expectations. Try to do a little more each day or each week and you will see steady progress. Strive for perfection but don't expect it every single day, or else you could give up out of frustration with yourself and the process.

Embrace Your Obstacles

As soon as you have goals, obstacles arise. Some you will be ready for; others will catch you off guard. This is a natural response to your efforts and should be taken as a positive sign. It means that you are challenging the *wall* around your *mindset*.

I know there's no such thing as a challenge free ride to your goal in this journey, but what separates us from reaching our goal? I want you to know, it's not the challenges nor the situations; it's not the conditions that you face along the way that stop you. It's the choices you make under those conditions that separate you from getting to goal or not.

It doesn't matter what happens to you, what matters is what you do about it! I learned that it's not the troubles, obstacles and problems along the journey that are so different; it is our solutions that vary. A lot of us dwell on the obstacles instead of working on solutions; that's understandable. The obstacles we face affect our thoughts and emotions as well as our results and cause us to question whether we are on the right track.

I want to tell you that, if you are being challenged, you are on the right track. If you persevere, all the headaches, hassles, frustrations and "transitional costs" in the short-term, it will be worth it. Do not shrink away from these obstacles, but find ways to win the battles and grow as a person. You have to focus on the solutions, not the obstacles. You will have obstacles, but with every obstacle there is a solution.

Challenges are not there to stop you; they're there to test you. When a challenge arises, the question is, are you ready for your goal this time? Are you serious this time? Obstacles are put in your way to see if your goal is really worth it to you. Is this your time? If you are ready, you will find a way; if not, you will find a way out.

At some point, you will hit a fork in the road of this journey. Have the unconditional commitment to your lifestyle change to see it through. When you hit a fork in the road, take it; pick up that fork, eat something healthy with it and move on!

Whenever you run into a *wall*, find a way around it; if not, learn how to knock it down (study until you learn how to). Once you stop fighting for what you want, what you do not want will show up. There will be challenges along the way, but they are there to test you, not to stop you. It's when you overcome these challenges that growth and learning occurs.

This is where you create your determination because you know you are doing the right thing. With each victory over your obstacles, you start to build momentum. With momentum, you build confidence, self-esteem and start to create new habits. Eventually, these habits become automatic and you create the lifestyle of the person you want to become. These are the moments you find out who you really are.

I have observed that my most successful clients, focus on finding solutions sooner than others. I urge you to practice this habit as well. These clients would create systems that helped them become better and work through their challenges more effectively. Having a plan or a system means that you make a conscious choice of how to respond effectively to the problem and then use this system each time the situation comes up.

For some, it could be eating a healthy meal before going to a party. For others, it could be planning in advance what to eat at the party. Find your own response to your problem areas and prepare your mental or physical cheat-sheet for each.

Remember, obstacles can stop you temporarily, but only you can stop you permanently. Just know that when you truly want to change, you will never give up, no matter how bad the situation may get. The challenges you face along your weight loss journey will only last temporary, but quitting will last forever. Never give up when you are faced with a challenge; show yourself you can do it.

Don't wish it was easier, wish you were better! Don't wish for less obstacles, wish for more solutions.

– Jim Rohn

Avoid Temptations

A lot of the fables and scriptural stories we heard as children, involved wise men being able to avoid the temptations that monsters and tricksters used to lure them into a trap. When you commit to a healthy lifestyle change, you will often find yourself in the shoes of these wise men.

Life sends a lot of temptations our way and it becomes our job to recognize temptation for what it is and stand firm in our path. It helps to have a plan ready for such situations as well. It is natural that you will be tempted by the old habits you had and a smart choice is to recognize that you will face these temptations.

Have an action plan in place. Doing so means that you don't have to forage for a response to the temptation; it will already be a part of your arsenal. Knowing what to do or say will give you the confidence needed to take effective actions and stick to the results you want to receive.

People who plan for obstacles are more likely to stick with their goals. For example, maybe your goal is to go for a walk every morning. What if you wake up one day and it's raining? Or you have an early morning meeting, which cuts into your exercise time? You may be tempted not to follow through. Have a back-up plan like, *If the weather's bad or I can't step out for some reason, I'll spend 20 minutes working out to a DVD in the house. I will spend 20 minutes walking up and down the stairs if I can't take a morning walk outside. I will either take an evening walk or exercise to a DVD in the evening at x time.* These solutions will help you stick to your new routine. Be specific about your alternatives in term of time spent, the effort taken and energy spent to ensure that your alternatives are as effective as your original plan of action.

Remember that you have the power to make a choice at every stage. Your choice can be one that is in line with your old conditioning or one that helps you develop your new condition. Initially, you may find that making the right choice is the hardest thing you have to do; you will slip up at times. But use these moments as learning experiences and find a solution that works for you. I promise you, with time, the choices become easier, the actions become more automatic and the new conditioning takes over and you will receive the results you want.

Avoid Comparisons

Comparisons happen all the time in the weight loss industry. We feel compelled when we start our own journey of weight loss to compare ourselves to other people who are also dieting or have already lost weight. I've seen how devastating this can be to your own results.

> ***Dieters – focus on other people dieting and get upset if they are not receiving the same or greater results.***

> ***Life changers – focus on their own experiences and know that everyone is different.***

Some people choose to share their journey to becoming healthier with a friend or significant other, in the hopes that each of them will be able to keep the other motivated during the low moments. But sometimes, one person starts seeing results faster than the other. This can be very disheartening for the person falling behind.

If this is you, it is important to avoid comparisons as much as possible. Remember, even though you are both journeying in the same direction, you each have your own journey. There are unique challenges that each person faces. Sometimes you will have an easier path and they will have a harder time. Sometimes it's the other way around.

Some of the factors that can influence the speed at which you make progress may be out of your control – like health issues or genetics. Remember that a number of subtle factors play a role in deciding how fast you progress on your journey. The goal here is to progress; as long as you are progressing, you are doing the right thing at your own speed.

Do not compare yourself to others. The only comparisons you should make are with your own past and future. Compare yourself to your starting point to see your progress. Identify points where you need to course correct and compare yourself to your goal state. This will motivate you to make additional effort. Each time you find that you are further from your starting point and closer to your goal, you will know that you are doing the work necessary to get there.

Plateaus

Nothing is more motivating than seeing progress, but what happens when you stop seeing those results?

When we make progress quickly, it feeds our emotions. Then, when there's a period of waiting or we hit a plateau, we find out how committed we really are and whether we're going to see things through to the finish or quit.

– Joyce Meyer

DOUBTFUL DIETING TO LASTING LIFESTYLE CHANGE

Hitting plateaus are a natural part of the weight loss process. Some people are lucky and see a consistent weight loss, but these are few and far between. For most, some rapid change is followed by a period where the body seems to be resisting efforts to lose weight. This can happen for a number of reasons.

After a time, our bodies adapt to our changed diet and exercise regimen; thus, we are less likely to lose weight. For others, the increased exercise can lead to feeling hungrier and thus more eating that they didn't account for. For some others, a medication may be interfering with their weight loss or there may be other reasons for interference.

Take a minute to evaluate if you have truly hit a plateau – if you have, try and understand the reason why. Be truthful with yourself about what you have been eating and any exercise that you have been doing (or not doing).

Dieters – think if the scale is not moving, the diet is not working and it's time to quit.

To them, numbers mean everything.

Life changers – plateaus are going to happen; if it continues, it's time to switch it up.

You can't dwell on how unfair it seems that the scales didn't go lower, but focus on how much weight you've already lost and keep going. If you were losing weight regularly and have more to go, and for no apparent reason you don't lose a single pound in over three to four weeks, it may be a sign that you have hit a plateau. A plateau does not mean that your regimen is not working; it just means that you may need to tweak your routine a little or change it.

Shake things up, switch it up and try a new exercise; increase exercise or try a new nutrition plan. Ensure that you are not eating more by comparing your meal journal entries across the weeks. Watch your portions and snacks as well as exercises. See what you want to switch up, but remember to keep it livable and sustainable.

Final Words

> *The only time you will never see results is by giving up. Refuse to give up. But if you tap into your motivation to persevere and stay flexible in your approach –*

There are many small and large potholes on the path to your new self. Your mind will rally against you; life will throw up tricky situations and temptations, and your body will adapt to your changes and slow your progress. But if you tap into your motivation to persevere and stay flexible in your approach - get curious, not furious with your results – you are destined for success. Use all experiences as opportunities to learn about yourself. Harness mistakes and turn them into the knowledge that informs you about the most effective strategies that are as unique as the individual you are.

Action Steps:

When you have already started on your journey towards your goal, a lot of roadblocks will come up. Use these action steps to keep you on your path:

Meal logs: Be diligent about maintaining a meal log. Knowing what and how much you eat and exercise will help you identify areas that need your attention. Also, the accountability of having to write everything down itself, helps you to control your diet/exercise more. This serves as a great piece of information to discover your patterns and habits when it comes to your health or unhealthy practices.

> Have patience, pay attention to your life experiences and write down what causes you to eat more or exercise less. See if there is a trend and respond by making a plan to effect change in these situations.

Learning from failure: Keep track of the points where you were unable to meet your daily goals. Understand what happened and then find a solution or solutions to the problem for the next time. Keep tweaking your plan with each learning experience.

Strive for 'Progress Not Perfection': Try to do better each day; not to be worried about being perfect every day. Compare how close you have come to your target each day and push yourself to do a little better every day and each week. Slowly, you will find yourself meeting your goals.

Embrace your obstacles: Obstacles will happen. Keep track of them, and when you find yourself challenged, evaluate what need has been triggered. Plan for them as much as you can. Study and learn from them and form responses based on the obstacles you are finding yourself running into.

Avoid temptations: Temptations are a natural part of the process. Recognize them when they come and try to avoid them when possible. If you succumb once, use that as a learning experience to formulate your response for the next time. If you can foresee them, have a plan. Either avoid the situation completely or fortify yourself so you are less influenced by the temptations.

Avoid comparisons: Use others' presence to motivate you; use inspirational stories from others to inspire you but avoid comparisons. Only compare you with yourself. Use others as support buddies to learn from and resist temptations. Remember that their journey, although parallel to yours, is different from yours. Your only comparisons should be to your starting point and your end goal.

Plateaus: Expect plateaus. Look out for them and use them as a marker for when you need to review your eating plans, meal journals and exercise habits. It may be time to tweak or switch up your routine.

Maintain For Life

#6. The Principles Of Maintenance For A Lifestyle Change

Congratulations!! At this point you are very close to your goal or have already achieved it. Give yourself a pat on the back and celebrate your successful journey.

For most people who lose weight only to gain it back, the biggest reason is because they operate from their old *mindset*. They hold onto unhelpful attitudes, philosophies and beliefs towards lifestyle, food and weight. This is what you have to be weary of. When I hear things like, *I can't wait until this diet is over so I can eat like I used to,* I know that person is in trouble. Their weight-loss is only temporary because they truly haven't changed their *mindset.*

Remember that the changes you have made are livable changes for a reason – you want to live with these new habits and choices for the rest of your life. People often fall into the trap of believing that their new actions and choices are applicable only until they lose all their excess weight. The moment they reach their goal, they promptly revert back to old behaviours that led them to gain weight in the first place. Do not fall into this trap – either because someone pushes you or because you relax your efforts.

If you have been following the process of this book, you have actually been thinking of maintenance the whole time. You have been preparing for this moment and for all the moments to come. You have made healthy changes that leave you feeling healthy as well as satisfied with your *mindset*, actions and body. Now you just have to keep doing the same thing and enjoy the new, fitter you for the rest of your life.

Don't let fear and doubt get the best of you! The tools that you learned, the habits you have formed and the healthy lifestyle you created, are going to change your life forever, if you allow them to.

Maintaining The New You

The course of maintenance frequently follows the same course as dieting. It's easier in the beginning, but at some point, it gets more difficult and then it gets easier again. Similarly, maintenance can be hard sometimes, but it will get easier as you strengthen your new habits further.

You are very close to having created a new comfort zone by now. Depending on how long it took you to get to maintenance, a lot of your old habits may feel distant and many of your new habits have become second nature. I'm sure you are still taking some conscious effort to practice the new healthy habits, but they are becoming more and more automatic. This in itself insulates you from gaining back the weight – your new comfort zone overtime will become as hard to break out of as your old one was, as long as you practice these new habits daily. And since this comfort zone is built on habits that are healthy, you will be more likely to make healthy choices in the future versus unhealthy. Remember, habits have buddies.

Preparing For Maintenance

There is something like a mourning period after you lose the weight and learn to let go of your old self. For many people, it takes time to accept their new selves. Sometimes, we are not fully ready to have this new body and be this new person. Subconsciously we sabotage our results and do everything we can to put the weight back on.

We remember our past conditioning and *mindset*. If you have followed this book closely on your journey, you will have learned to let go of the old *mindset* and the past way of thinking. You will have to become more comfortable in this new self.

At the same time, you know that at the core, you are still the same person with the same basic values. The only beliefs, attitude and personal philosophies that have changed are the ones about your health, food and exercise.

When you lose weight, you cannot hide it; you are a walking billboard. You will get attention from your peers and family, because of your change, and they will ask you how you did it. People are going to look at you and talk to you about it; this can be hard for some people, especially those who don't like to be the center of attention.

You may also find that some of your friends or family may treat you different or may expect you to revert back to old habits now. Just be aware that some people are not ready for your life change. This can create pressure for you to fall back into old ways of thinking and old habits. Recognize this, if and when it happens. Remind yourself of why you started this journey and why you saw it through. Remember what you have learned and recognize the joy your new choices, new habits and your new body have given you.

Buffer Weight Or Weight Range

Now that you have reached your goal, you can relax a little. You still have to push yourself to practice the habits and choices that brought you here, but you can give yourself some flexibility. At the same time, do not stop practicing your healthy eating habits and exercise behaviours; they are essential to maintaining the new you. You still need to exercise regularly, eat healthy foods and sensible portions that brought you to your goal – all while still paying attention to how you respond to external and internal pressures.

I find that one thing that happens to a lot of people when they reach their goal, is that they relax completely and stop doing all the things that got them to that point. When this happens, the weight goes up quickly. When it starts to creep up, a lot of people fall under the trap of saying/thinking, *well, I know what to do to get this off, so I can take it off whenever I want.* But unfortunately they never do, because past habits come back and take over their new routine.

As you know, maintaining a precise weight is an illusion; you have to aim for health, not an arbitrary number. To this end, give yourself a buffer of 5 pounds near your goal weight. This is the range within which you should be comfortable with changes in your weight. Maintenance involves practicing healthy behaviours that will keep your weight in this range. But what I usually say in seminars and presentations is, why do you need a scale when you have pants? Now why would I say that? Because your pants will never lie. They will tell you if you are going up in weight or not. If your pants fit when you are at your goal weight, then start to get a little tight, you know it's time to revisit and reexamine your healthy lifestyle practices, and to get back on track.

Sometimes your weight will go up a little; sometimes it will come down a little, depending on the events happening in your life. Use this buffer to ensure that you do not lose too much weight or gain too much either. If you cross your buffer, you know that you need to change something. But fluctuation within this range is part of the natural process of maintaining a healthy weight and lifestyle.

Continuous Learning: Goals Are Never Ending

The key to maintenance is to know that reaching goals is both an end and a start. The most important part of reaching one goal is to use that as the starting point for another. As you become better at what you are doing, keep challenging yourself and growing. For example, to stay active, you could learn a new sport or try another new form of exercise. You could eat new and exciting things or try different ways of cooking and preparing healthy foods.

Being healthy is to dedicate yourself to learning continuously – about the needs of your body, about healthy foods and activities and about how new things affect your health. Being healthy does not mean being wary of new food and preparation. Being healthy means understanding them, understanding portion sizes and finding new recipes and options that are healthy as well as interesting to you. This way, you can keep things exciting while focusing on your health. Instead of getting into another boring rut, allow yourself to find new healthy goals and choices to add to your repertoire.

After I first lost weight, it started to creep back over the next couple of years. I realized that it was time to switch things up and try something new. So I started to look for new ways to keep me on track. At this point, both my father and I were hitting the gym regularly and I had already completed my education in nutrition. It was my father who asked me to devise an eating plan for us that would enable us to participate in a bodybuilding show. This was his idea of taking it to the next level. Although I had never thought about participating in bodybuilding shows as an option before, I jumped at the idea of sharing this goal with my father.

At that time, my 60+ year old father lost over 80 lbs for a show; I found a passion I never knew I had. It was a great way to motivate each other and we had a great time together working towards this goal. We were the first father-son duo to compete at the show.

While my father placed third in his class, he placed first in my eyes as he was the oldest participant in the show and did such a great job in preparing and dedicating himself to the process. I ended up placing first in that provincial competition and then went on to win my class at the Atlantic Canadian Championships that year. But our real victories were the shared experience, the added fitness and the new passion we both found for bodybuilding; we both competed in several others since.

We no longer compete in that many shows, but the point is that you don't have to take it to that level. It's whatever journey works for you, as long as you continue growing yourself, pushing yourself and finding new and healthy ways to continue to work, the process will work for you long-term.

Giving Back

Surprisingly, or not, one of the best ways to stay passionate is to pass the torch to someone else. Pass on your story when someone asks you how you lost weight. Tell them about all your challenges and all your choices. When you inspire someone else, you get inspired all over again. When you motivate someone, you get motivated as well. When you teach, you learn.

The more you live this healthy lifestyle, the more it gets contagious and the more people are going to ask you how you did it and for your secret. Share the ideas in this book with others. You can feel great when you look at the new you in the mirror, but you will feel truly fulfilled if you can help others do the same.

Never push your new lifestyle on anyone; they will push back. The people who truly want to change and are ready, will come to you. This is where you have a chance to really help someone change their life.

Another reason why talking about the process helps with maintenance is that, each time you talk about your journey, you think of it afresh. Each time you recount the details, you get in touch with the effort you have taken and learn to appreciate how far you have come. By talking about your success, you are also owning it and this will help in maintaining it.

This is your "story" now – tell it, show it and help as many people as you can do what you have done. Not only will you pass on the lessons you have learned, but you continue to learn and grow as a person as well. Give back.

Mindset Shift For Life

At times, your past *mindset* may still come to taunt you. Accept it as a reminder of your starting point and then use your new skills to return to who you are today. Occasionally you may find this difficult. But, as time passes, it will get easier until your lifestyle and routine is like muscle memory – an automatic response where you snap back.

Sometimes people regain the weight because they forget to practice what they have learned. Others succumb to weight gain because their environment always pressures them. Even if this happens, do not lose heart. You have done this once before and you can do it again. Remember the process – make good choices, focus on consistency, motivate yourself and ensure that you take action to get the results.

If you make the committed choice to change your life this time, it means that you are making the decision yourself. It means that you are taking 100% responsibility and are changing your rules and taking action. You know what to do to get focused and to focus on the right things. Ask yourself the right questions and use supportive internal language to maintain focus.

Pay attention to the process, find the right solutions and emphasize supportive thoughts over destructive ones. You know now that you chose the meanings to your emotions; how to maintain your motivation by always re-assessing and re-evaluating your goals, vision, beliefs, and your why. Take action until you get the results you want.

All it takes is a little effort and a little patience. I recommend that you read this book at least twice a year, or more, as repetition is key to a new *mindset* and to keep you on track. This will also trigger evaluation and appraisal of your lifestyle and any changes that you may choose to make to fine tune your healthy lifestyle.

Take yourself through all the action steps at regular intervals, just to keep your mind set for success and habits fresh and supported. The more you practice, the more you will find yourself doing everything we have discussed and without much thought.

Action Steps:

Celebrate your success: Pat yourself on the back.

Preparing for maintenance: Take a long, hard look at what steps you need to take to maintain your new weight. Recognize that you have made lifestyle changes, which means that you are still paying attention to how you treat your body. Understand that your weight will fluctuate naturally and accept a range within which your weight will fall.

Continuous learning: Find ways to keep your food and exercising interesting. Try new exercises, learn new recipes and try new healthy foods. Learn different ways to enjoy healthy living. Join exercise groups or a new class; find new activities and foods that excite you.

Giving back: Pass the knowledge on. Be assured that your own motivation and awareness will only increase each time you inspire someone else. Help and support someone going through the journey. This will also loop back and motivate you to maintain your new lifestyle.

Stay in touch with these principles and action steps. Use them to keep you on track and to fine tune your lifestyle when needed.

Final Words

The first section of this book gave you the information you needed to create an awareness of what holds you back from making a long-term change, and to build an understanding that YOU can make a lifestyle change. Also, we discussed and the importance of making lifestyle changes over crash dieting.

In the second section, we discussed the fundamentals and the principles that gave you solutions and necessary changes in the way you think, feel, choose, and act. We discussed the value of choice and committing to your goals and the factors that help you stay motivated. We discussed the importance of being focused, actions to take, and how to examine your results. We talked about what happens when you reach your goals and how to maintain your health and wellness.

As a part of each chapter, you also found a series of action steps. Some of you may have started working on these steps immediately; others may have chosen to first read the whole book and then start your journey. In either case, I urge you to follow the action steps very seriously. These are practical, focused actions that will help you identify your strengths, define your goals and keep you on your path. Eventually they will enable you to maintain your new healthy lifestyle.

As you practice these steps regularly, you will notice that you have changed the way you think about your health, food and fitness. You may also experience a change in the extent to which you feel motivated by different factors and in the way you respond to different situations. You will find yourself a cognitively and emotionally stronger person; a more confident one and a more positive person as well.

Keep going back and use these action steps as you feel the need. I truly enjoyed giving back to you – sharing the knowledge that I learned to help you make permanent changes in your life. Remember to always stay ambitious about being nutritious and to never give up!

THANK YOU

I want to personally thank you for taking the time to invest in yourself, and in your life. Now that you have thoroughly read and digested this information, I hope that you:

- are aware of your own reasons for eating.

- have made sense of why your lifestyle is what it is and how it contributes to your over all health and weight.

- have a path, or are closer to a path, for making the lifestyle changes for your unique set of circumstances.

Remember, it is not the lack of information that is out there about eating or exercising that causes failure. Take this blueprint and apply the principles taught to achieve optimum health through permanent, functional and sustainable lifestyle changes.

You will have to change the way you think about your health, and your life in general, if you want change. It starts with an idea, the idea that you are going to change your life. Then you must emotionalize this idea to lead to consistent actions. You must first work on the inside for the results you desire on the outside. Remember, it's not *what* you do for a week or a month – it's what you do *daily* that matters. The secret to success is found in your daily routine.

If you are asking yourself, *can I really do this, can I change my life?* If you don't believe you can, sometimes you need someone's belief in you before yours kicks in. I'm speaking to you from experience and from thousands of clients of mine that have used these principles and changed their life, that YOU CAN to. I believe in you.

Thank you for allowing me to be your personal transformational health coach in your journey to a healthier, happier you.

If you would like to continue your journey with me, you can contact me at www.devinleblanc.com.

Michelle Arakgi

Made in the USA
Charleston, SC
29 December 2016